ANESTHESIOLOGY

for kids

Medical School
FOR KIDS™

First paperback edition October 2022

Book design by Betty Nguyen & Brandon Pham

ISBN 978-1-957557-07-6 (paperback)

Printed in the United States of America

Published by Black Phoenix Press

www.mdforkids.org

To the friends and family who have supported and loved us unconditionally, and to the mentors who have guided and taught us more than we could have imagined:

Thank you.

Betty & Brandon

Medical School
FOR KIDS™

Anesthesiology

(a-nuhs-thee-zee-AA-luh-jee)

the branch of medicine concerned with the total perioperative care of patients before, during, and after surgery

Medical School FOR KIDS™

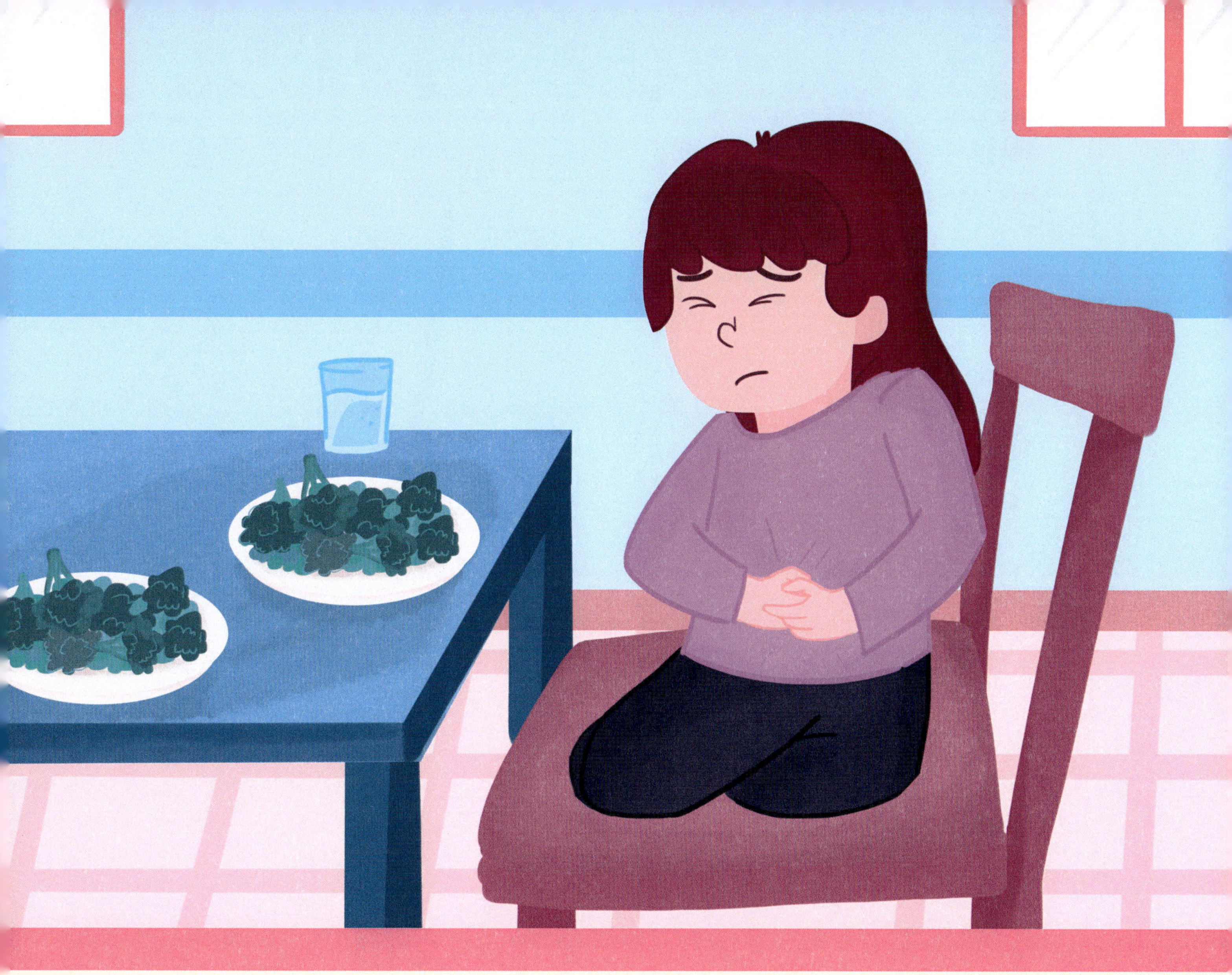

When we get sick, different parts of our body might start to hurt. This is called **pain**.

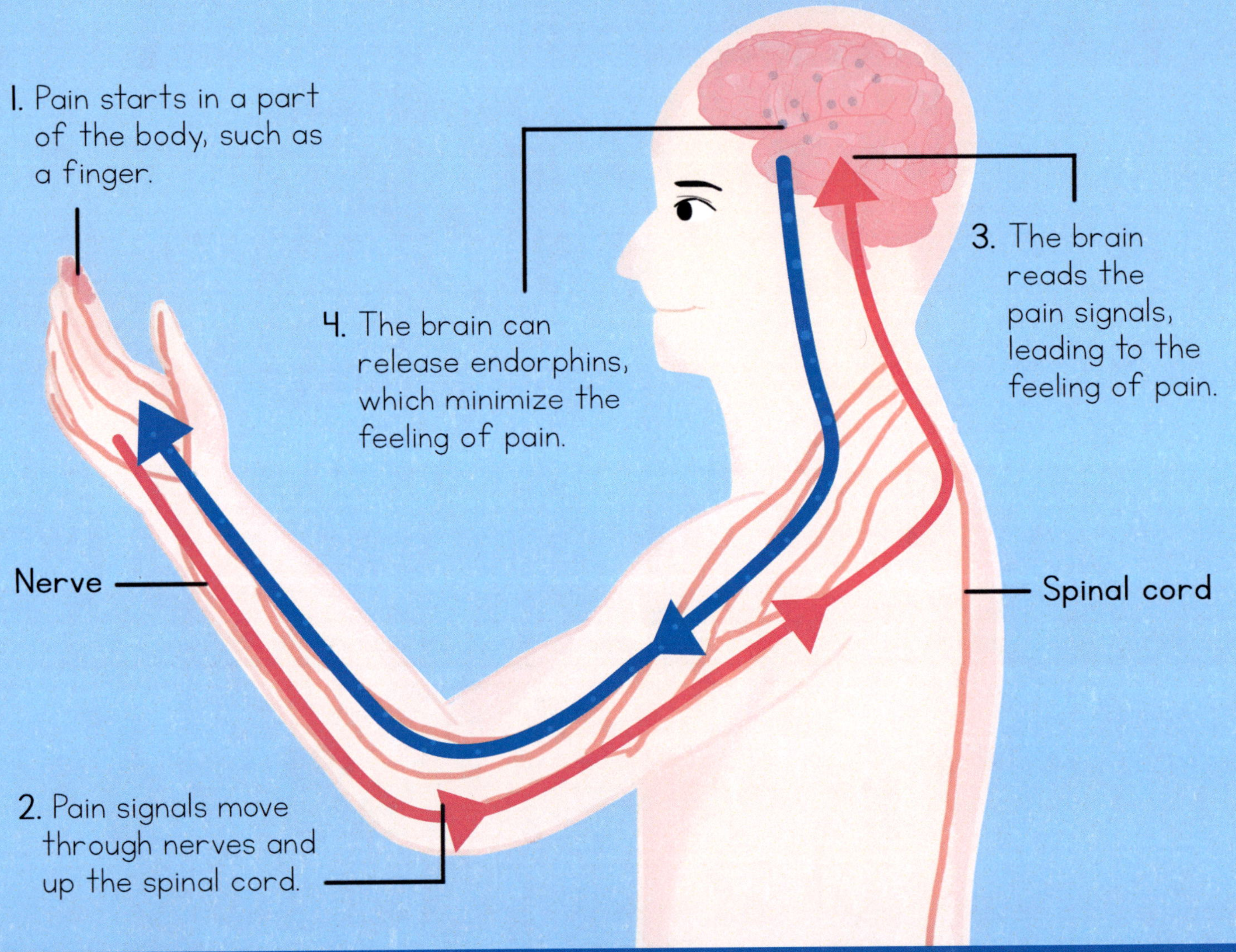

Pain is how our body tells us that something might be wrong. Pain signals travel from our nerves through our spinal cord to our brain.

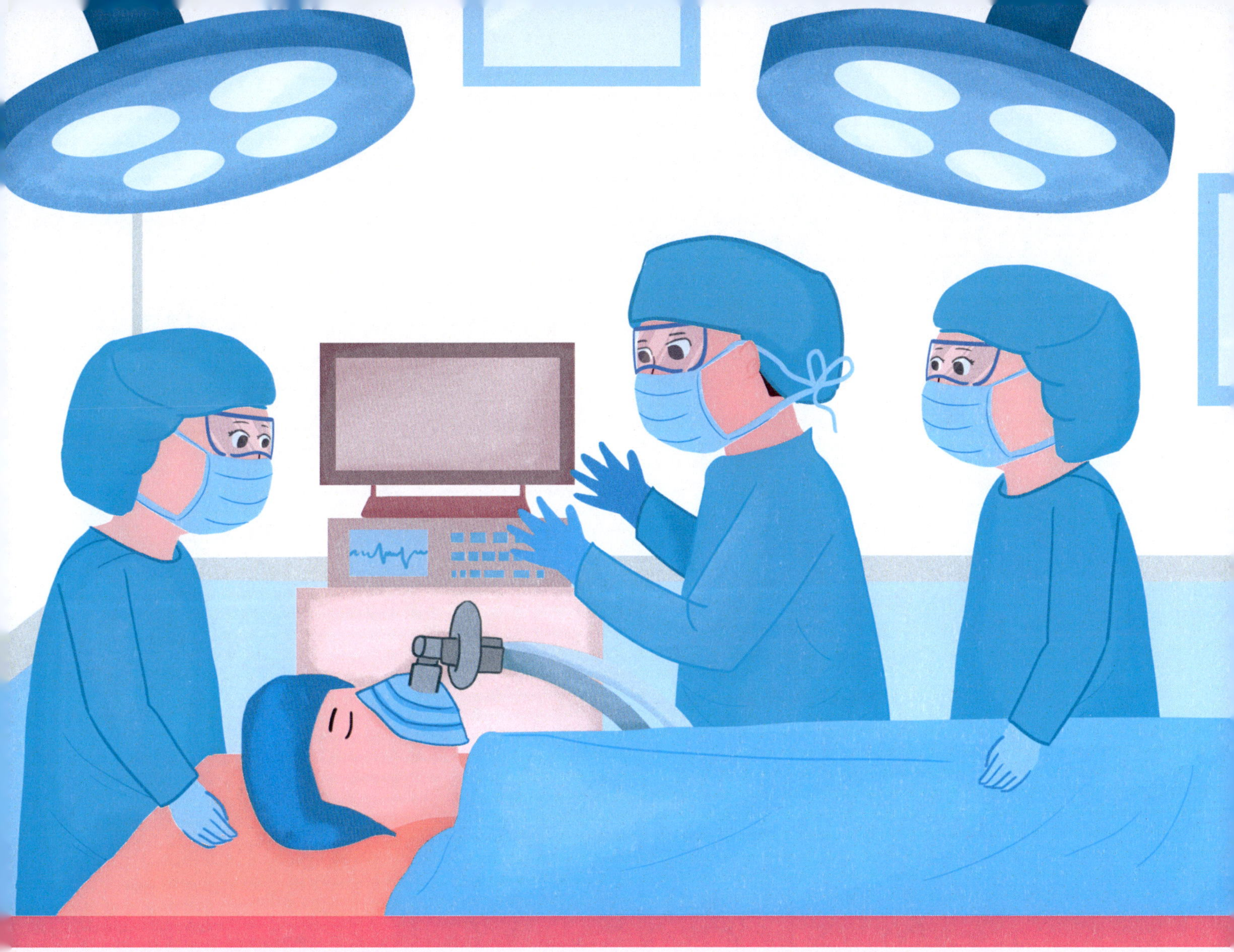

Sometimes, we need surgeries to treat certain medical conditions, but these procedures can also cause pain.

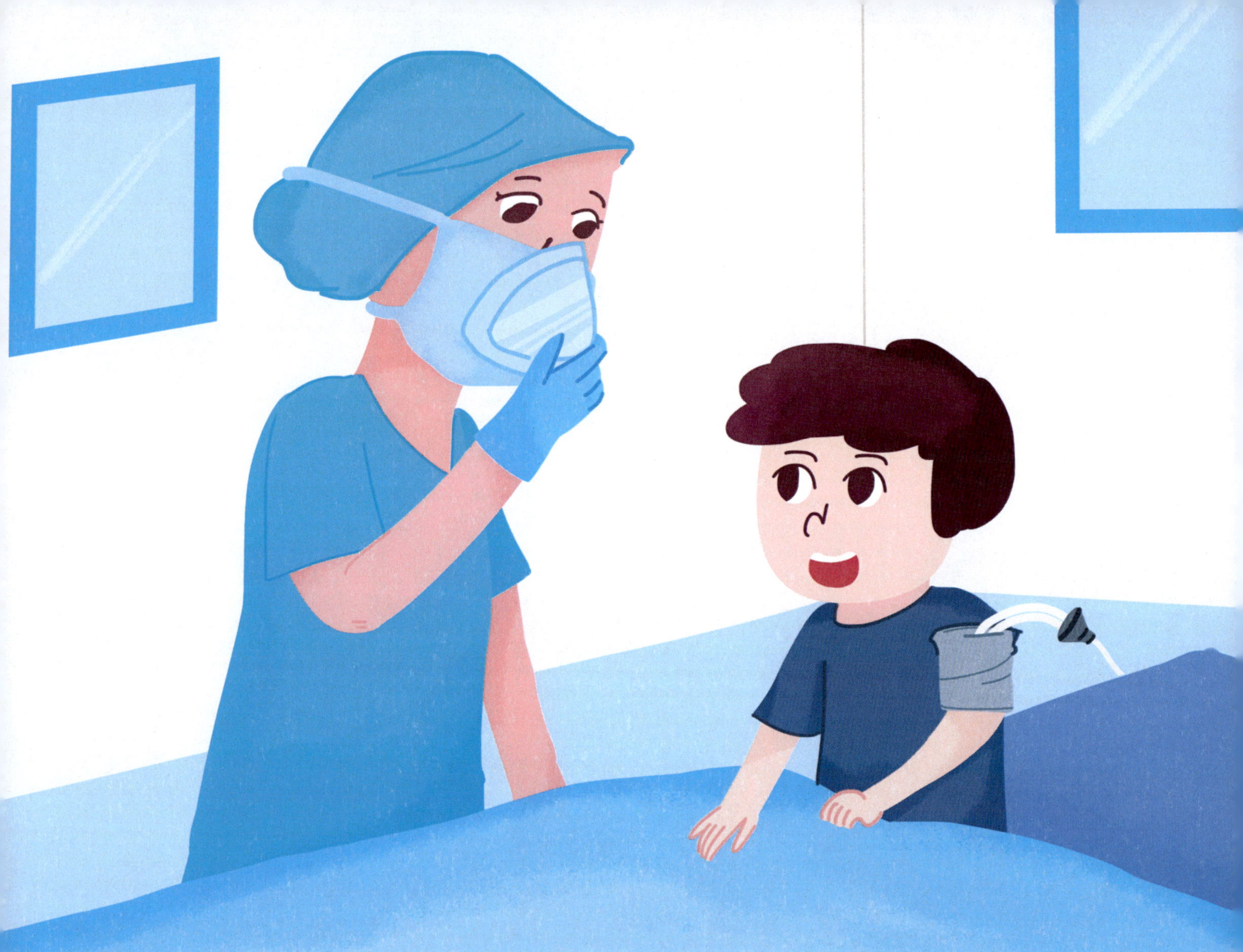

Doctors called **anesthesiologists** can give us medications that prevent us from feeling pain during surgery.

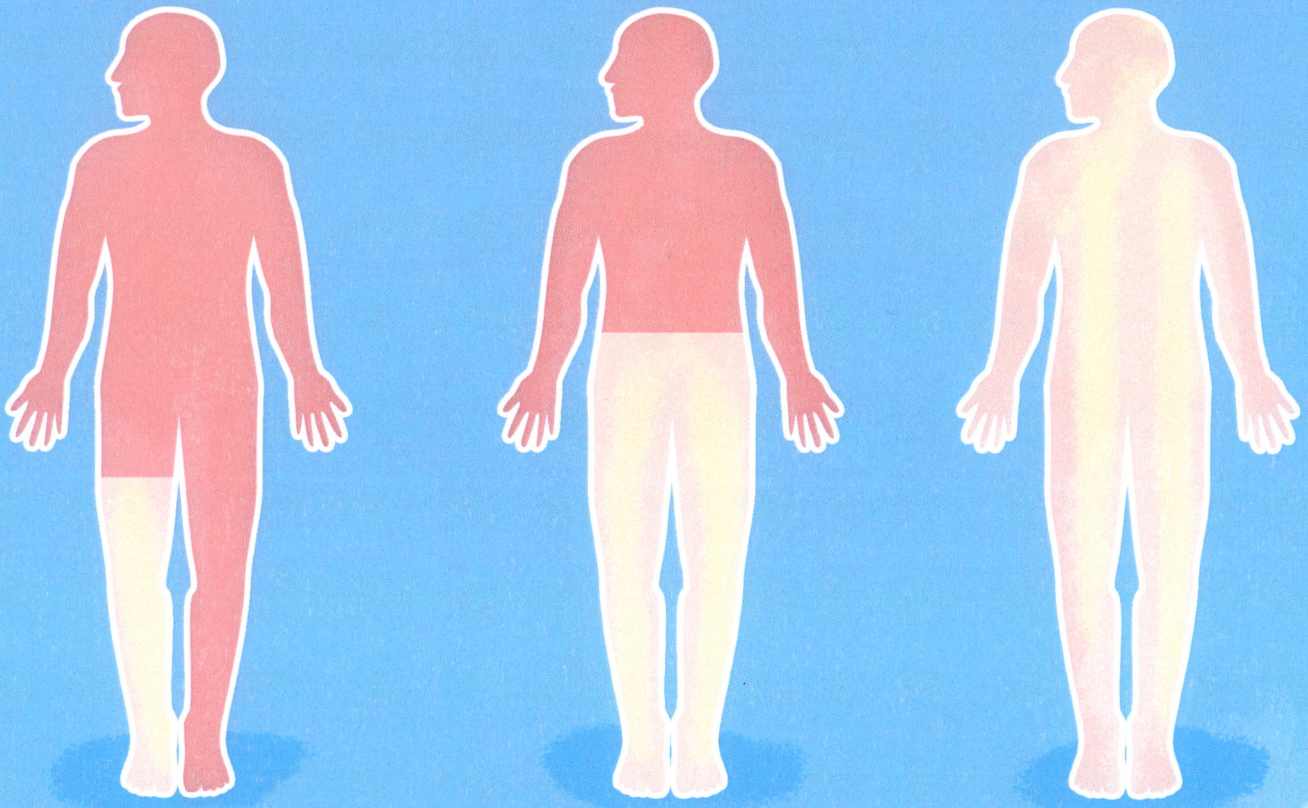

Local anesthesia

Causes loss of pain sensation to a **small part** of the body

Regional anesthesia

Causes loss of pain sensation to a **region** of the body

General anesthesia

Causes loss of pain sensation to the **entire body**

Anesthesia is a type of medication that blocks pain signals from getting to the brain. There are three main types of anesthesia.

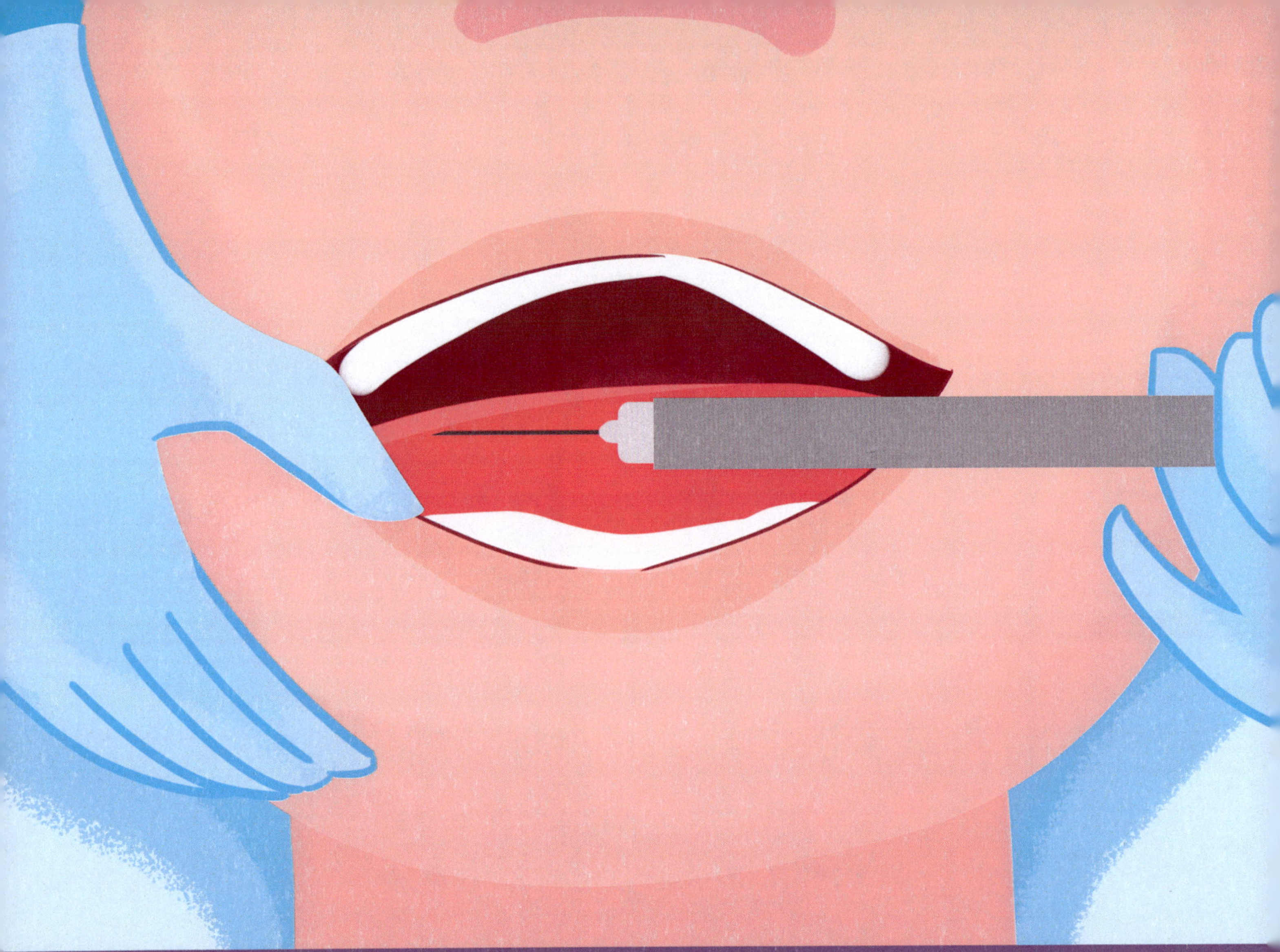

Local anesthesia numbs a small part of the body, like the hand or mouth. It can be given as an injection, spray, or ointment.

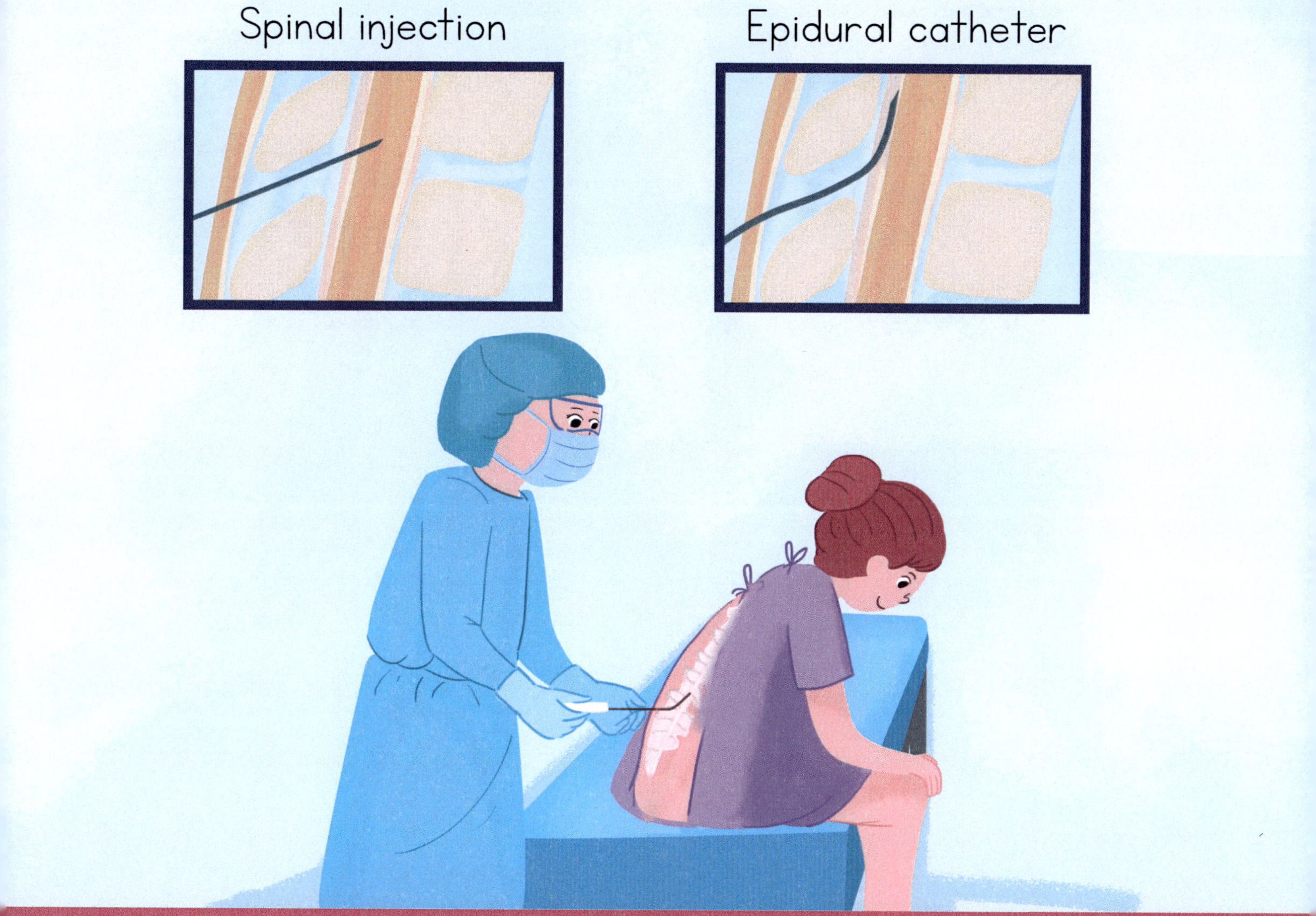

Regional anesthesia numbs a larger region of the body. It is given as an injection near a cluster of nerves in the spine.

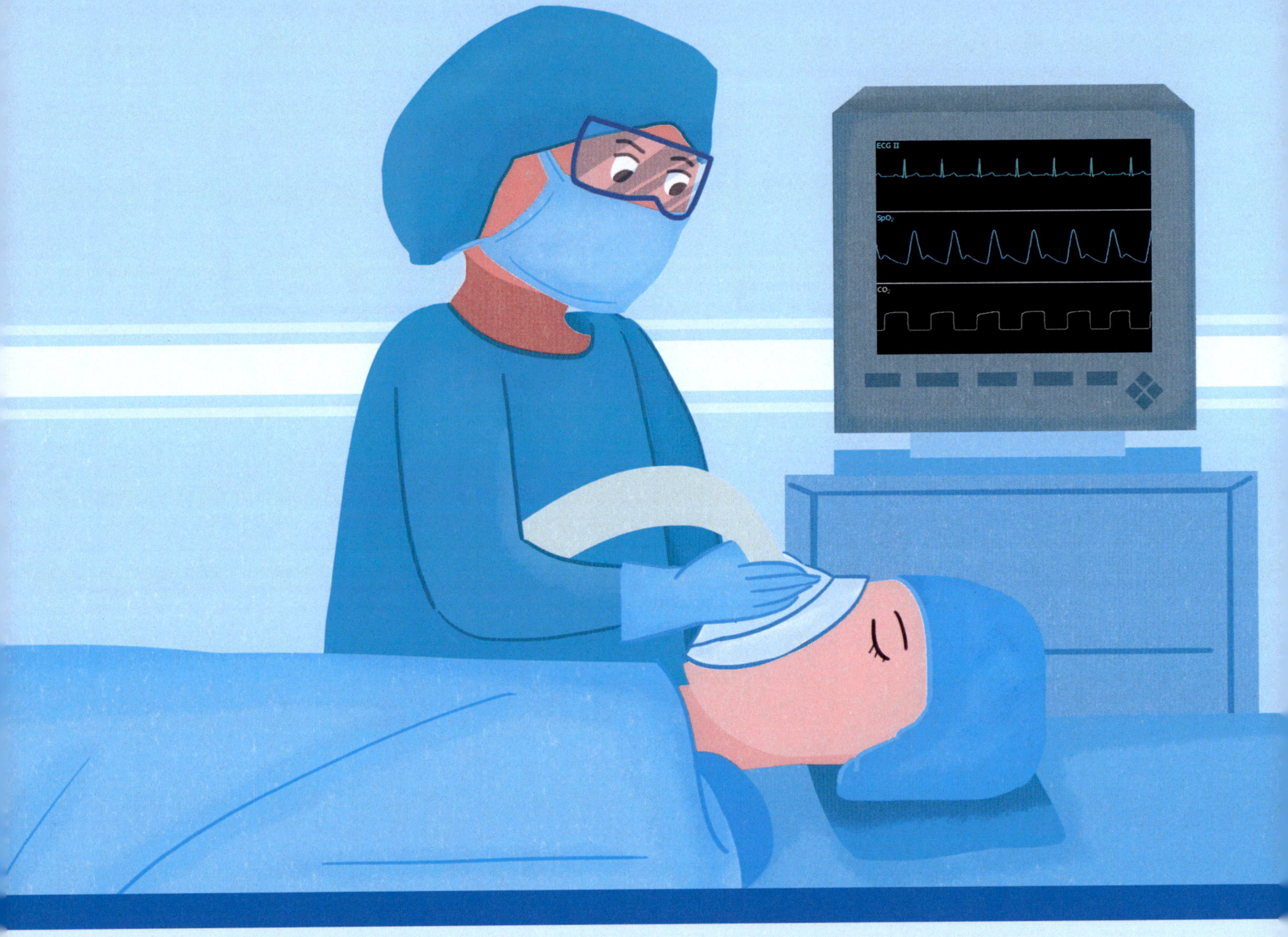

General anesthesia makes someone completely unconscious, or "asleep." It is given as an injection or inhaled gas.

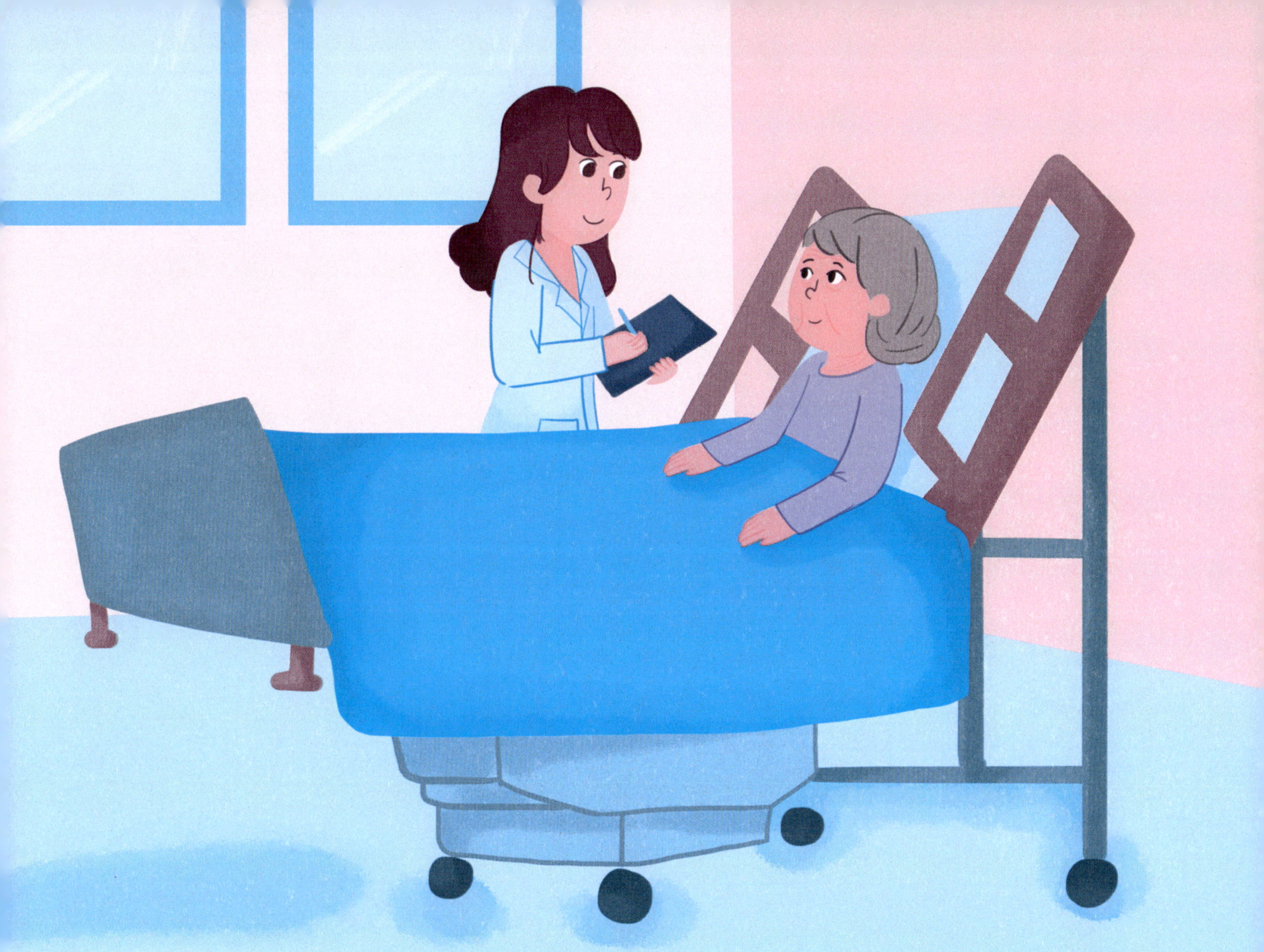

People of any age might need surgery. If you ever need surgery, knowing what happens in the hospital can help you feel more at ease.

Why You Can't Eat or Drink Before Surgery

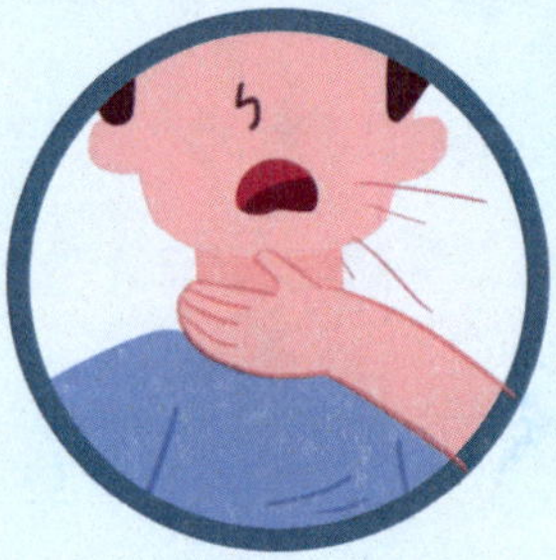

Risk of aspiration

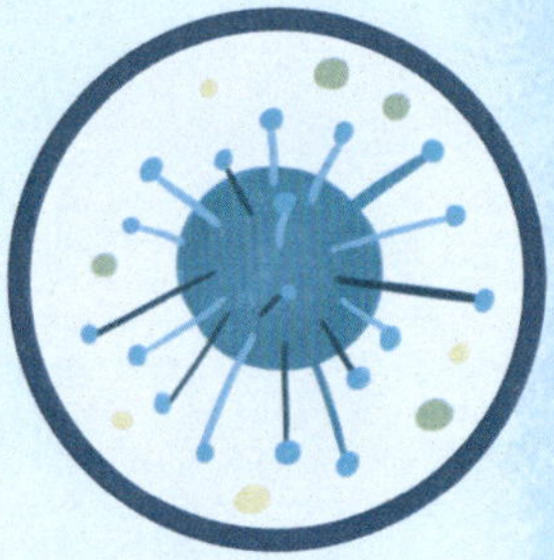

Risk of infection

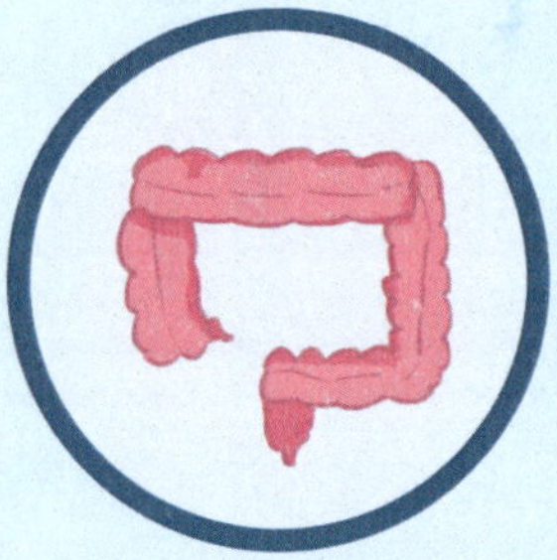

Bowel prep interference

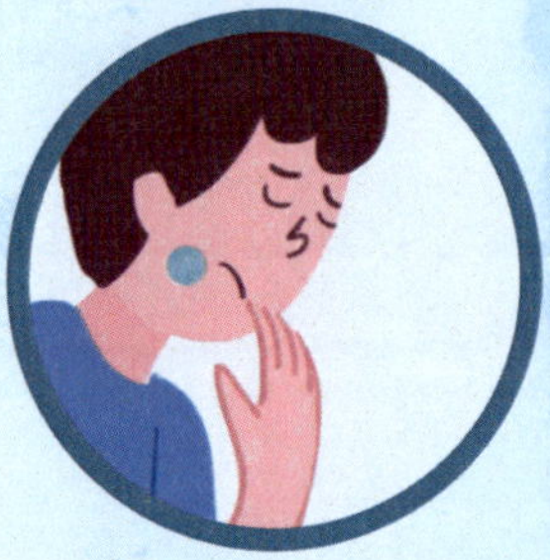

Risk of nausea and vomiting

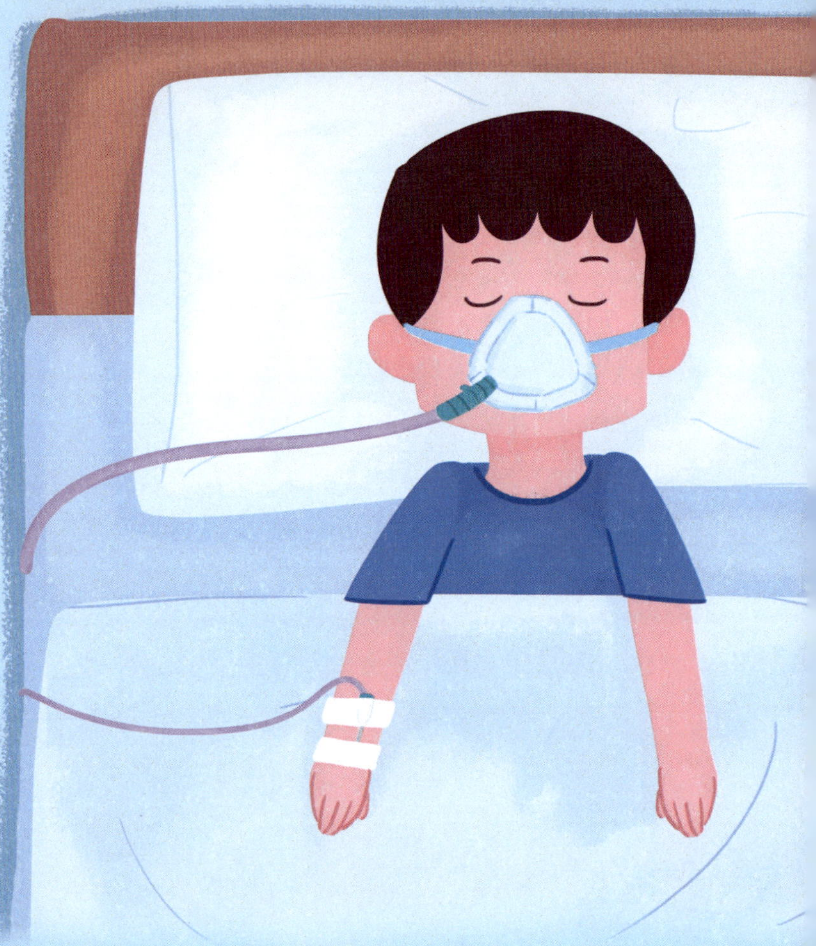

If you will be getting general anesthesia, remember that you will not be able to eat or drink before surgery.

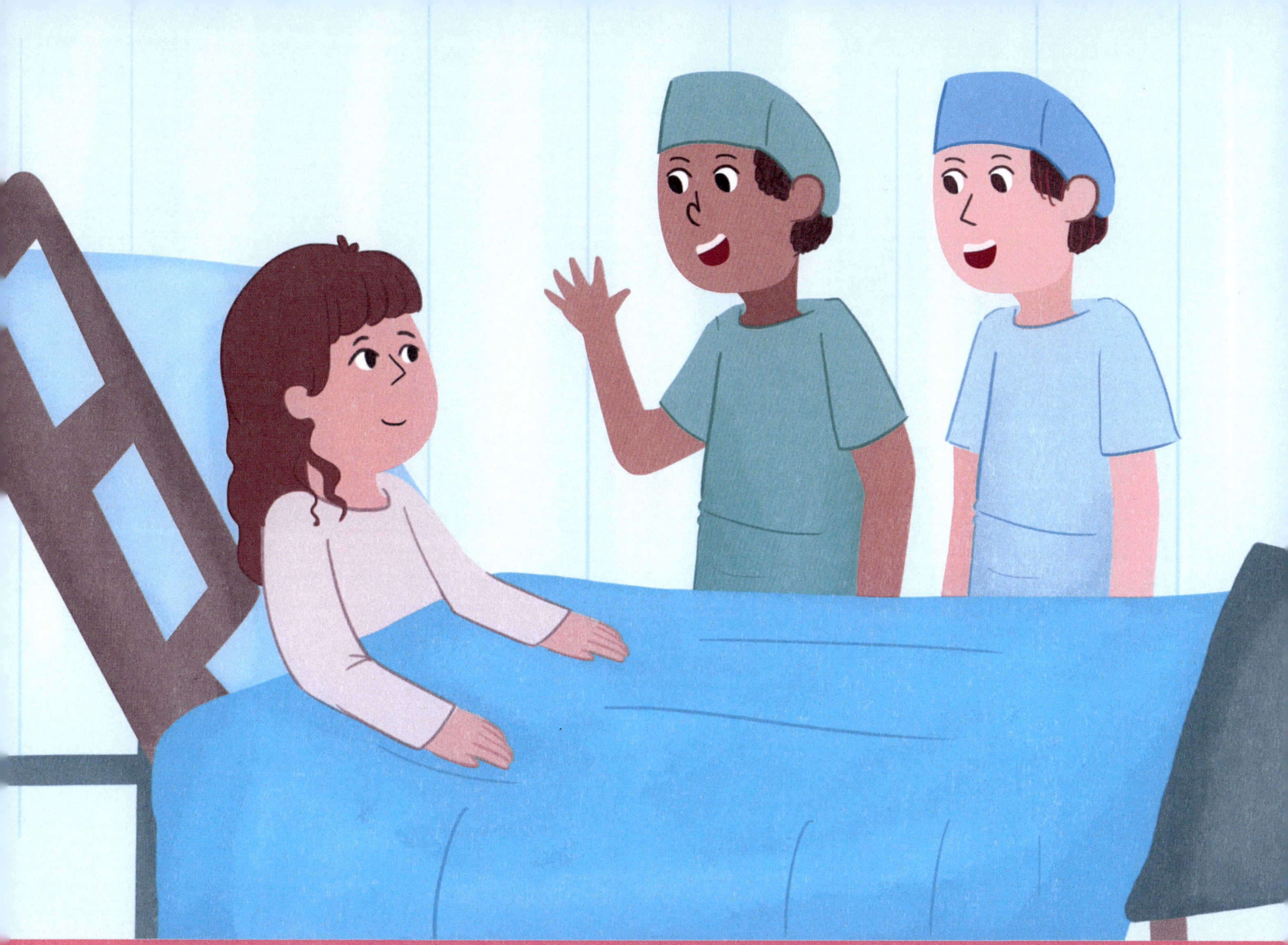

Before surgery, you will probably talk to your anesthesiologist and **surgeon**. The surgeon is the doctor who will be doing the surgery.

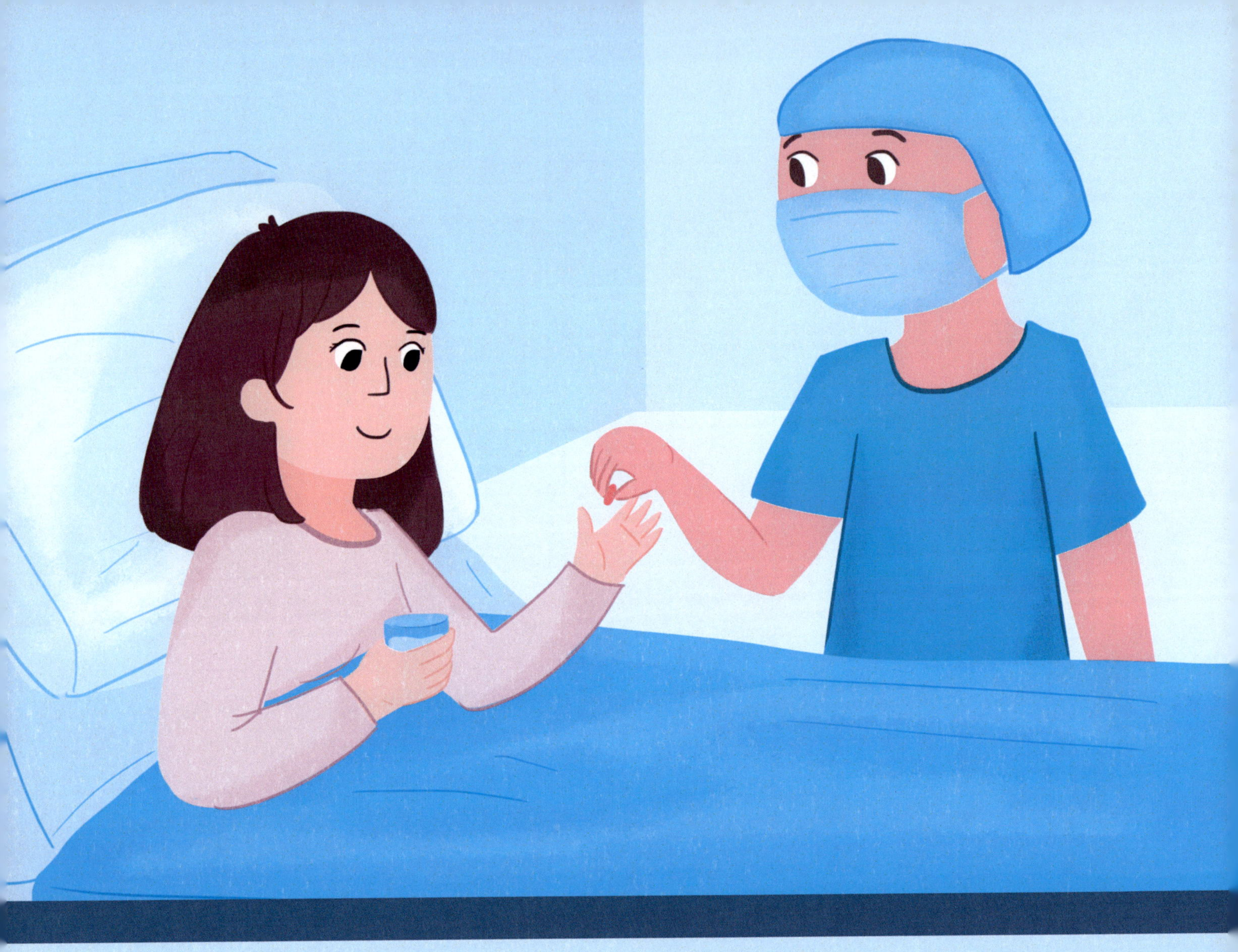

Surgery can be scary, so the anesthesiologist might first give you a medication called an **anxiolytic** to help you stay calm.

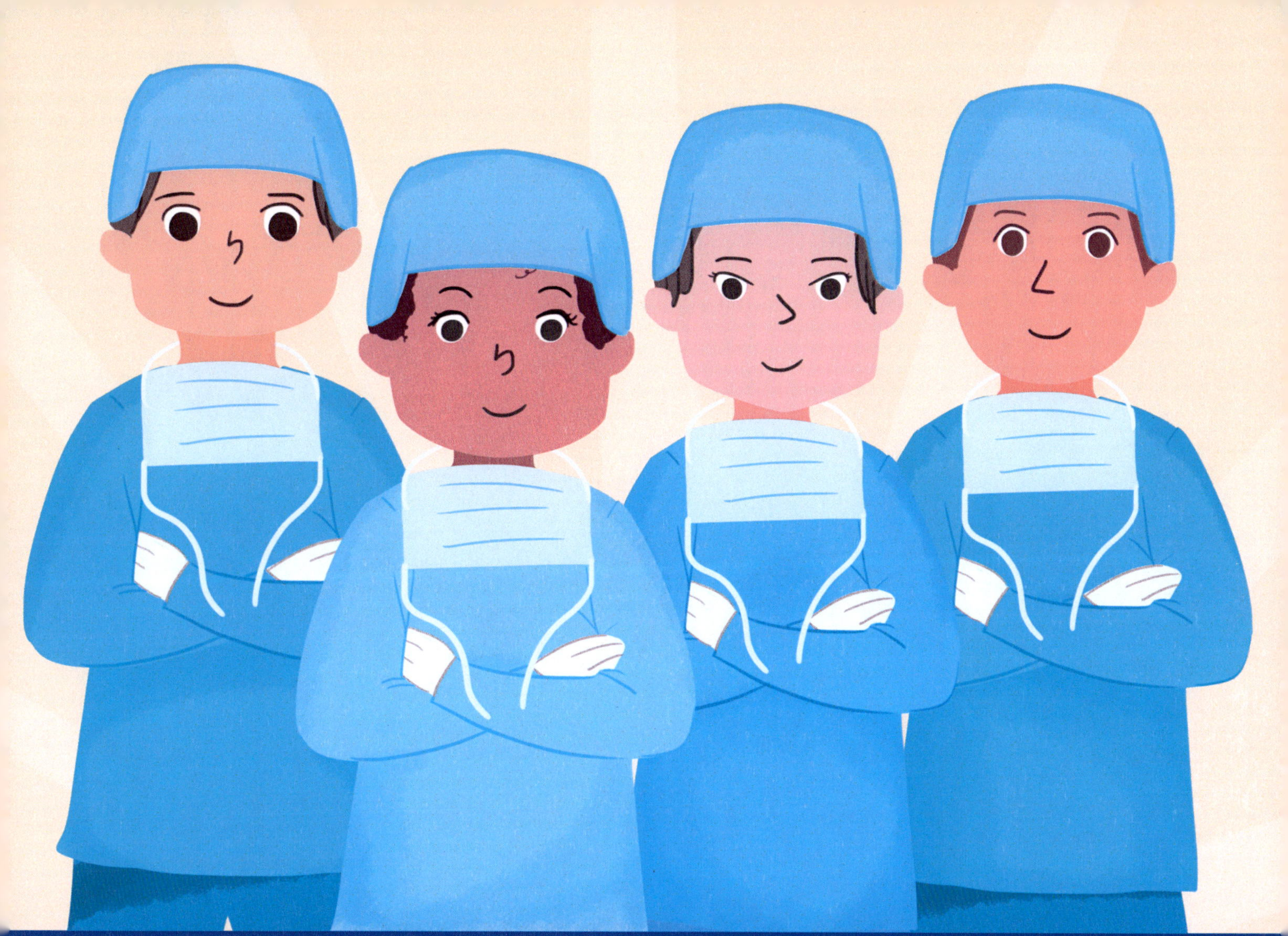

When you get to the operating room, you will meet many new people. These are nurses, technicians, and doctors there to help you.

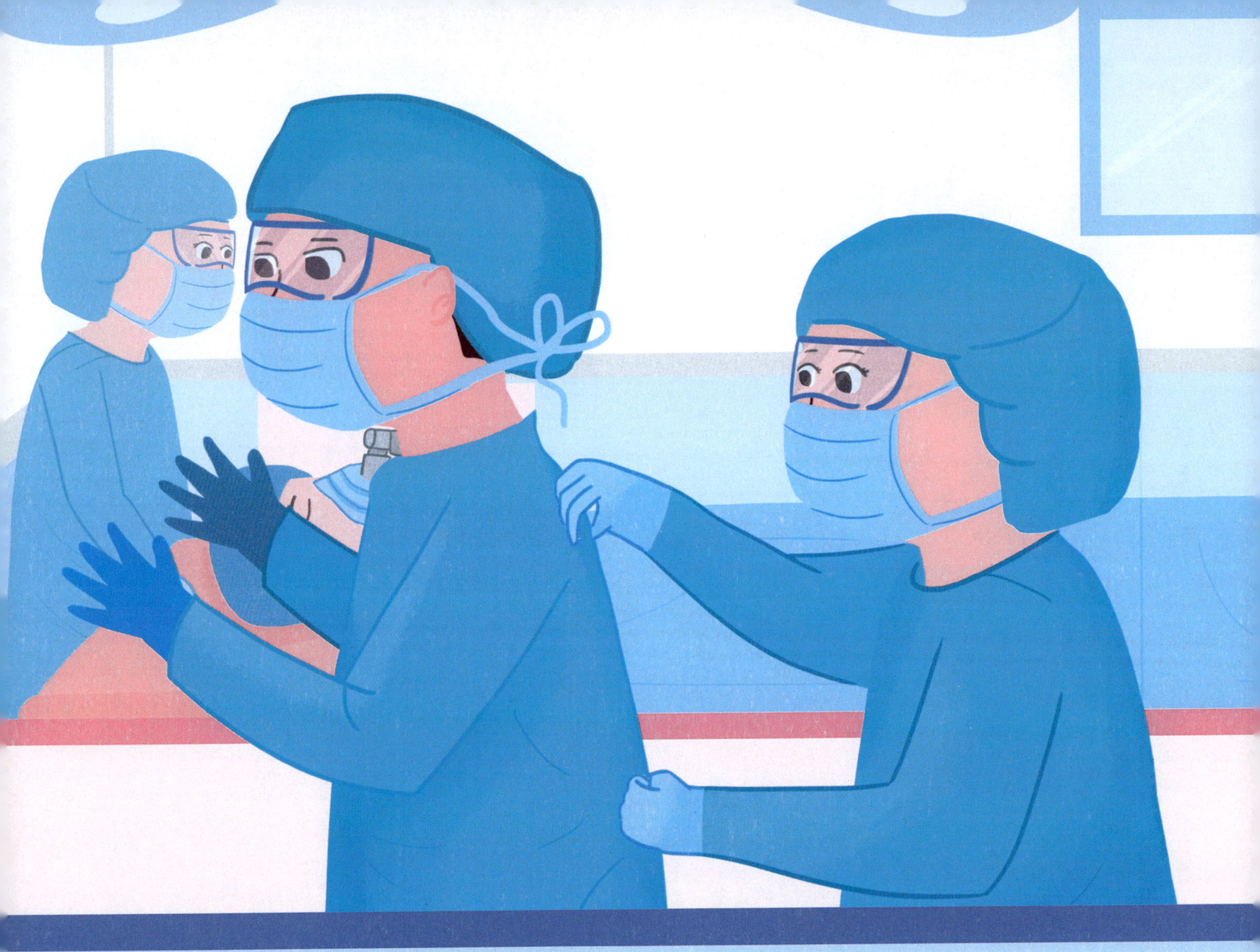

Everyone will be wearing caps, masks, gloves, and gowns to prevent them from spreading germs to you during surgery.

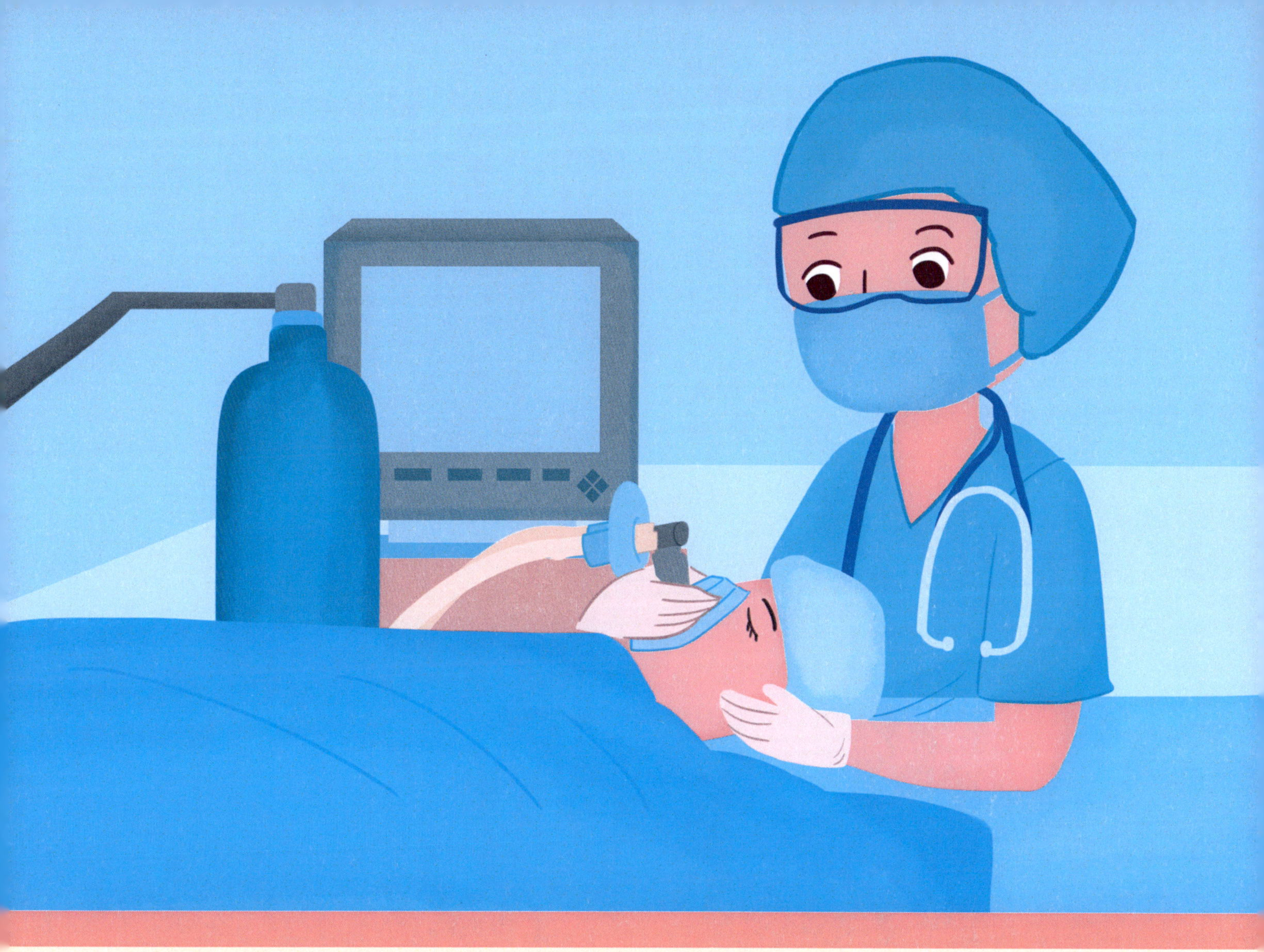

After the anesthesiologist gives you general anesthesia, you will fall asleep! You won't remember anything from surgery.

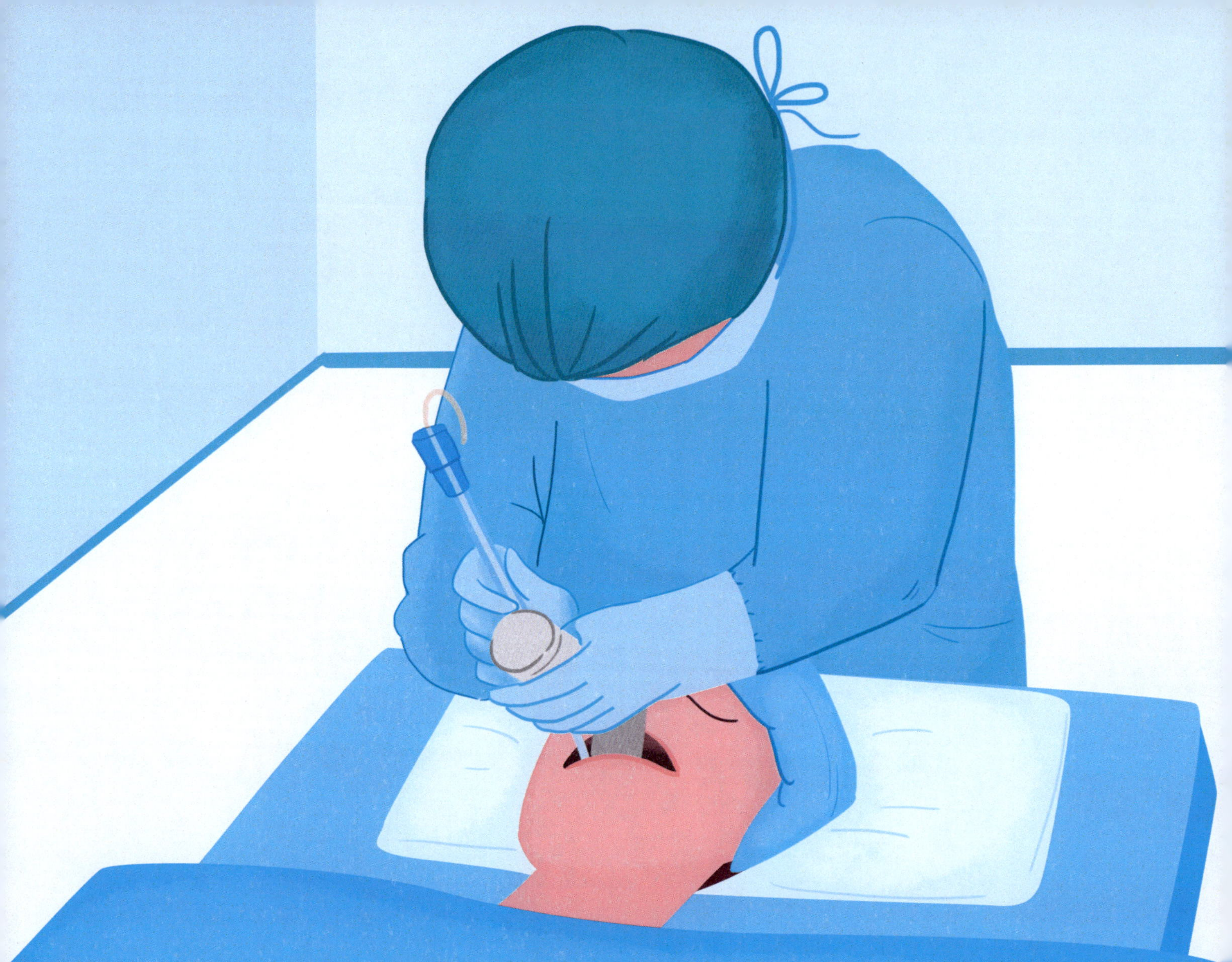

The anesthesiologist might place a tube in your throat to help you breathe during surgery. This is called **intubation.**

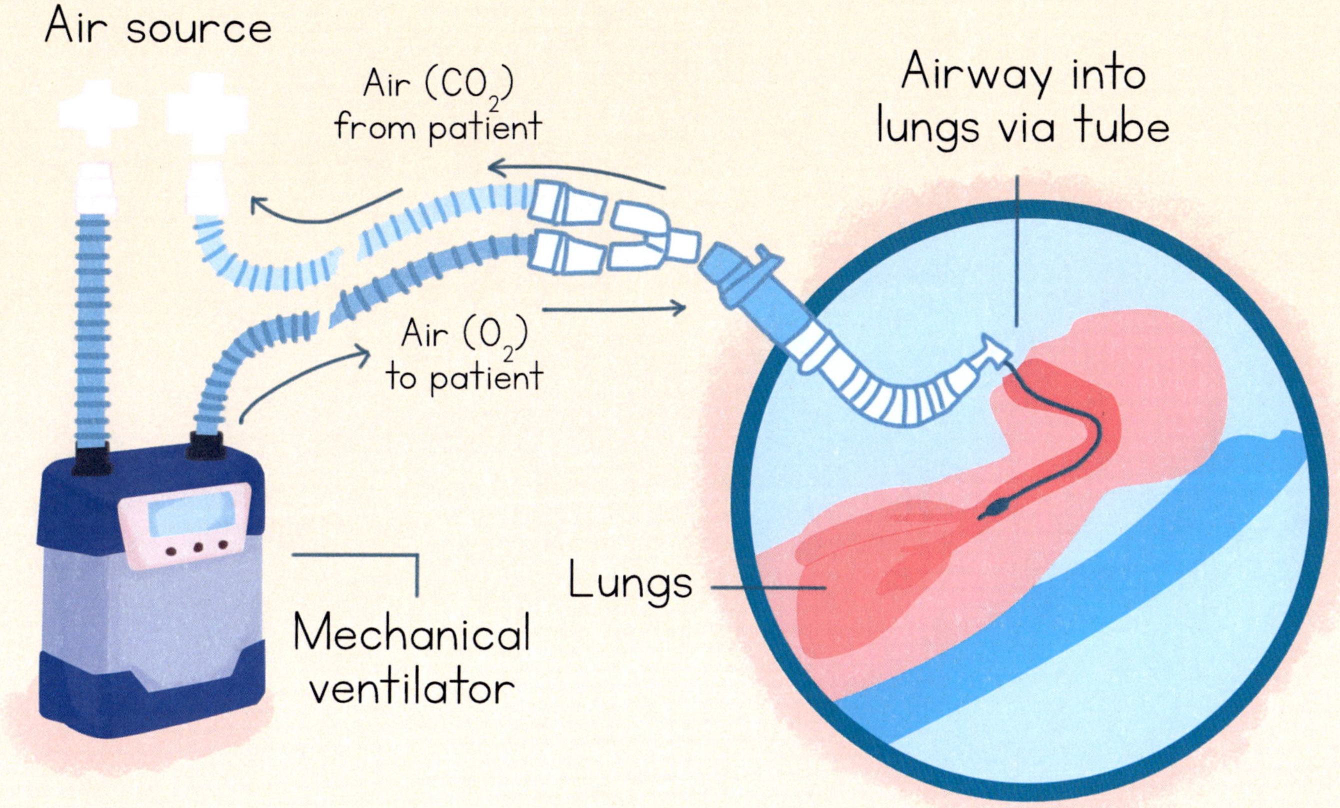

The breathing tube is connected to a machine that helps you bring air in and out of your lungs. This is called **mechanical ventilation**.

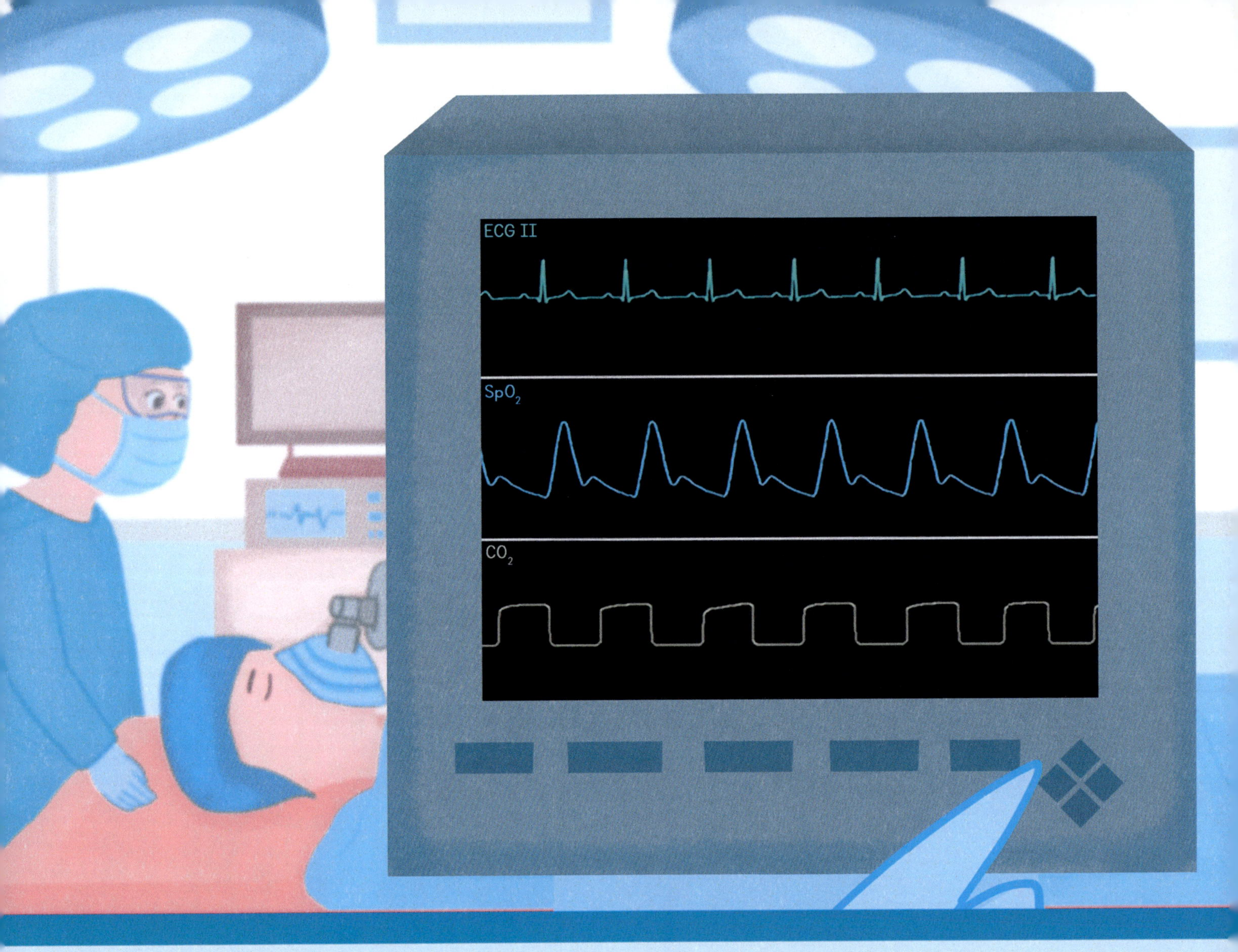

During surgery, the anesthesiologist works with the surgeon to make sure your **vital signs** remain stable.

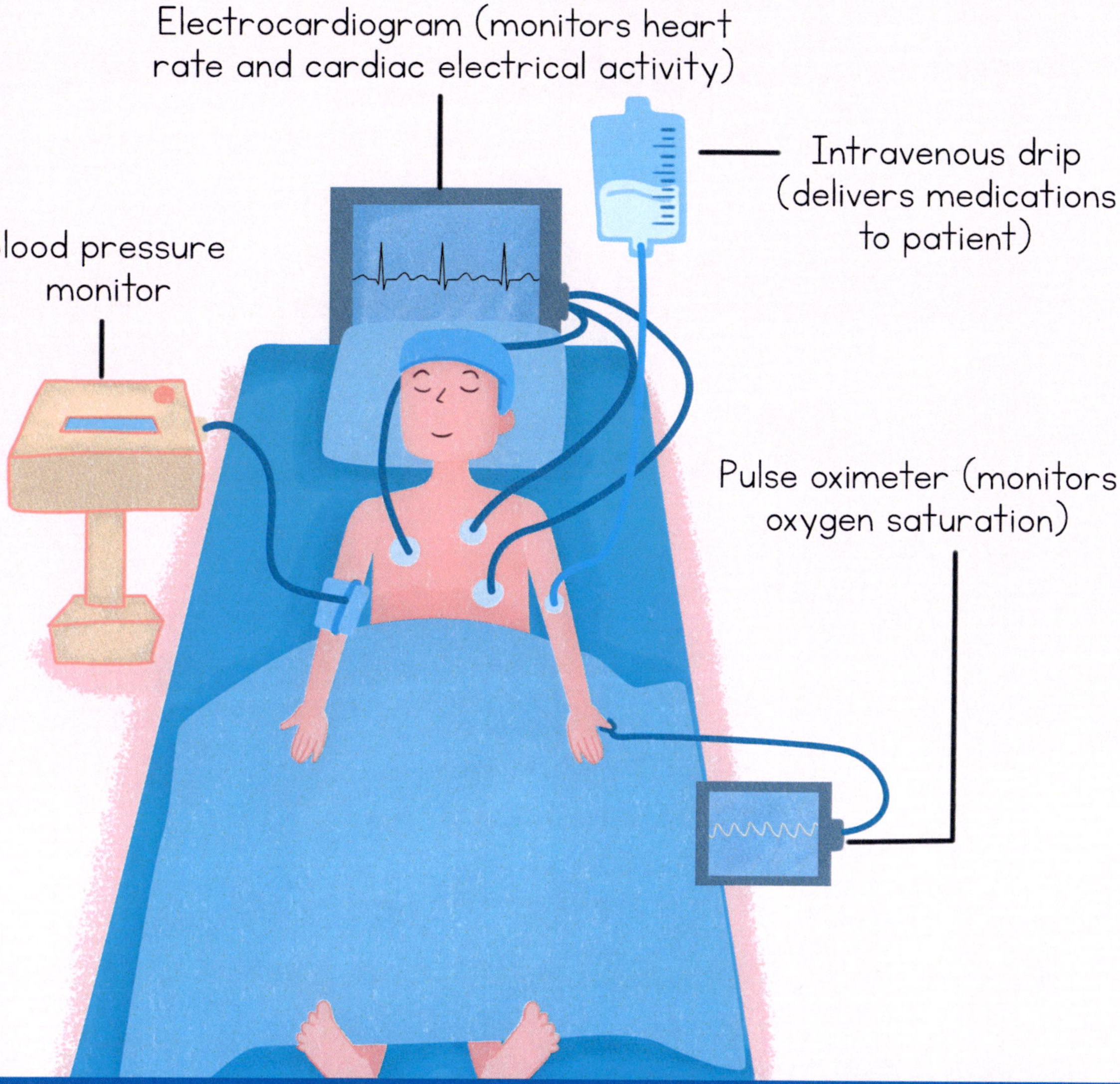

Your vital signs, such as temperature, heart rate, and blood pressure, show how well your body is working.

Post-Anesthesia Care Unit (PACU)

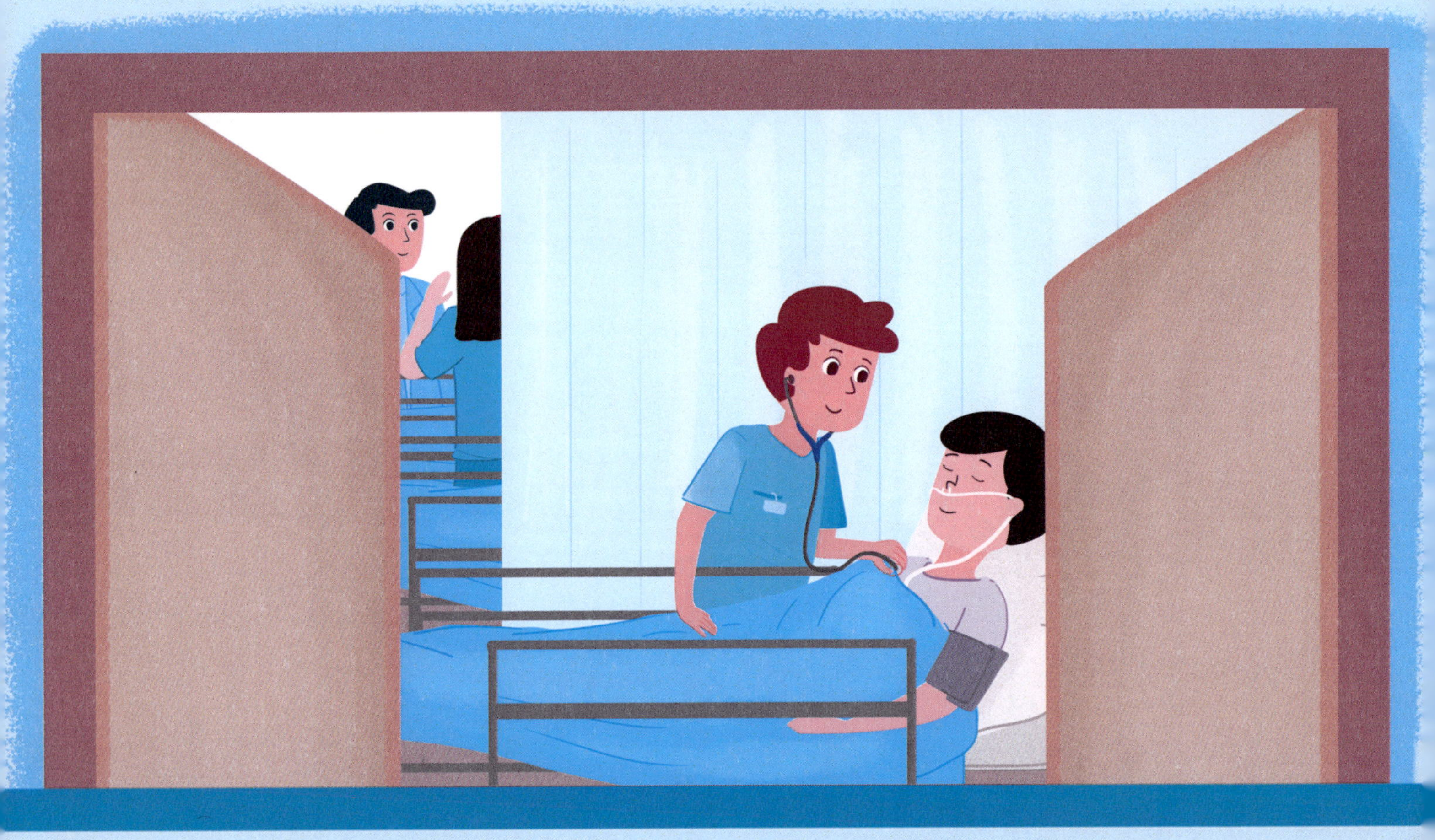

After surgery, the anesthesiologist will remove your breathing tube, and you will go to the **post-anesthesia care unit** (PACU).

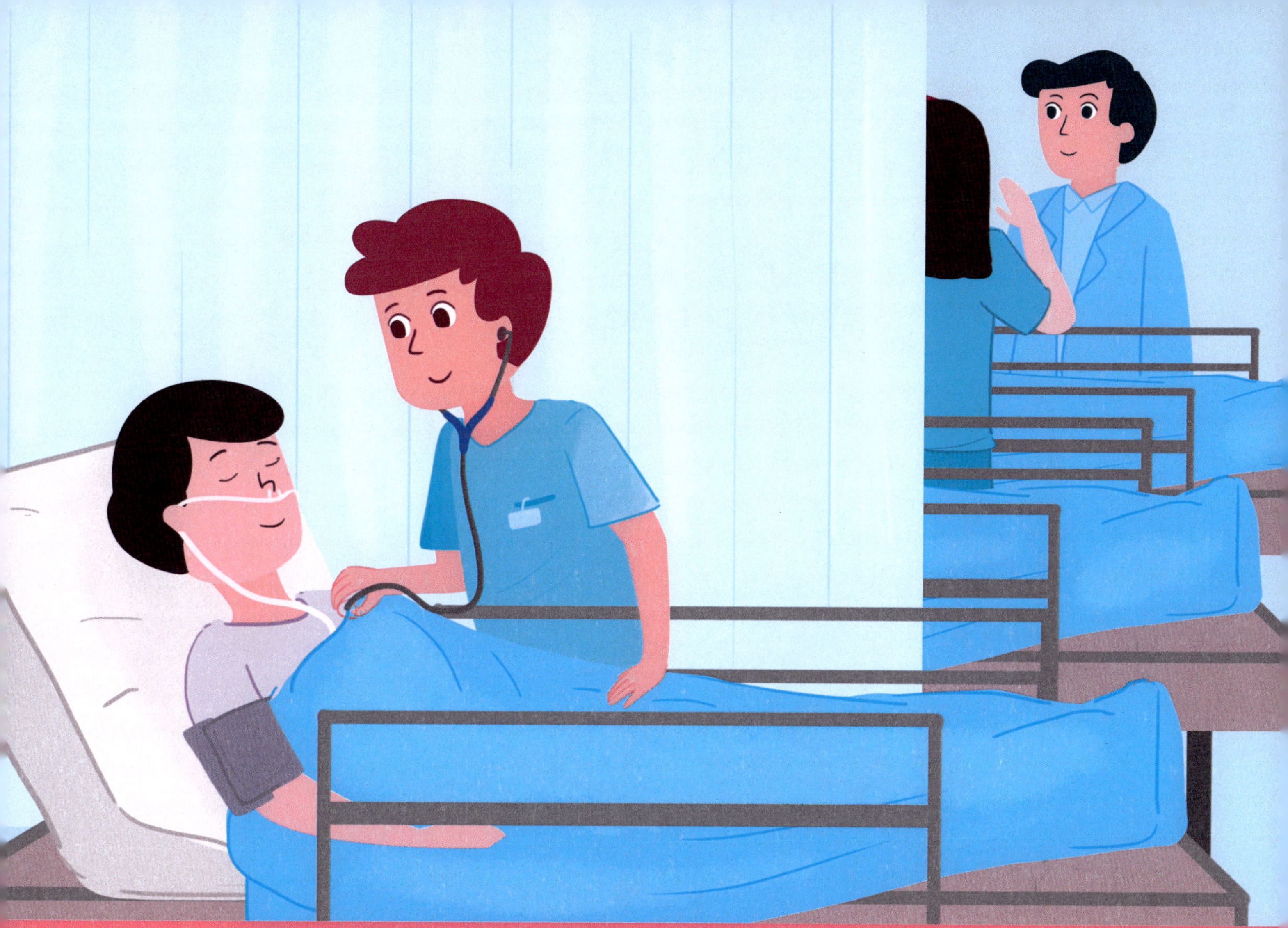

A nurse will be in the PACU to monitor you while you wake up. There will probably be other patients around waking up from surgery, too!

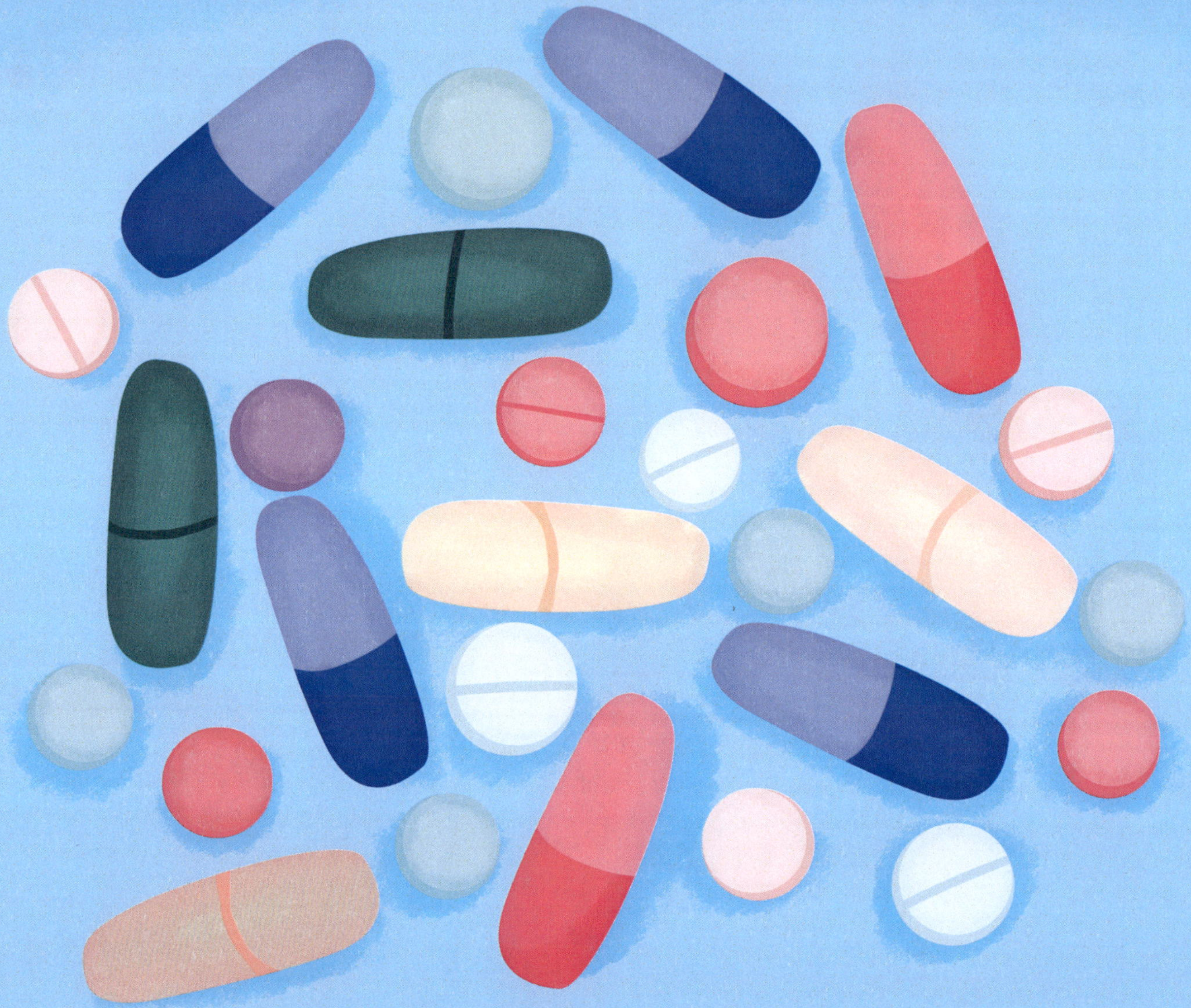

After surgery, it is common to feel pain. There are many different types of pain medications you can use to feel better.

		Ibuprofen	Acetaminophen
1	What type of medication is it?	Anti-inflammatory (NSAID)	Analgesic, antipyretic
2	What does it treat?	Pain, fever, inflammation	Pain, fever
3	What forms does it come in?	Tablet, capsule, liquid	Tablet, capsule, liquid, rectal suppository
4	What are the side effects?	Stomach upset, dizziness, heartburn	Rare
5	What organs does it affect?	Stomach Kidneys	Liver
6	Can you alternate them?	Yes	
7	How often can you take them?	Every 4-6 hours	

Ibuprofen is a type of non-steroidal anti-inflammatory drug (NSAID). **Acetaminophen** is another type of pain medication.

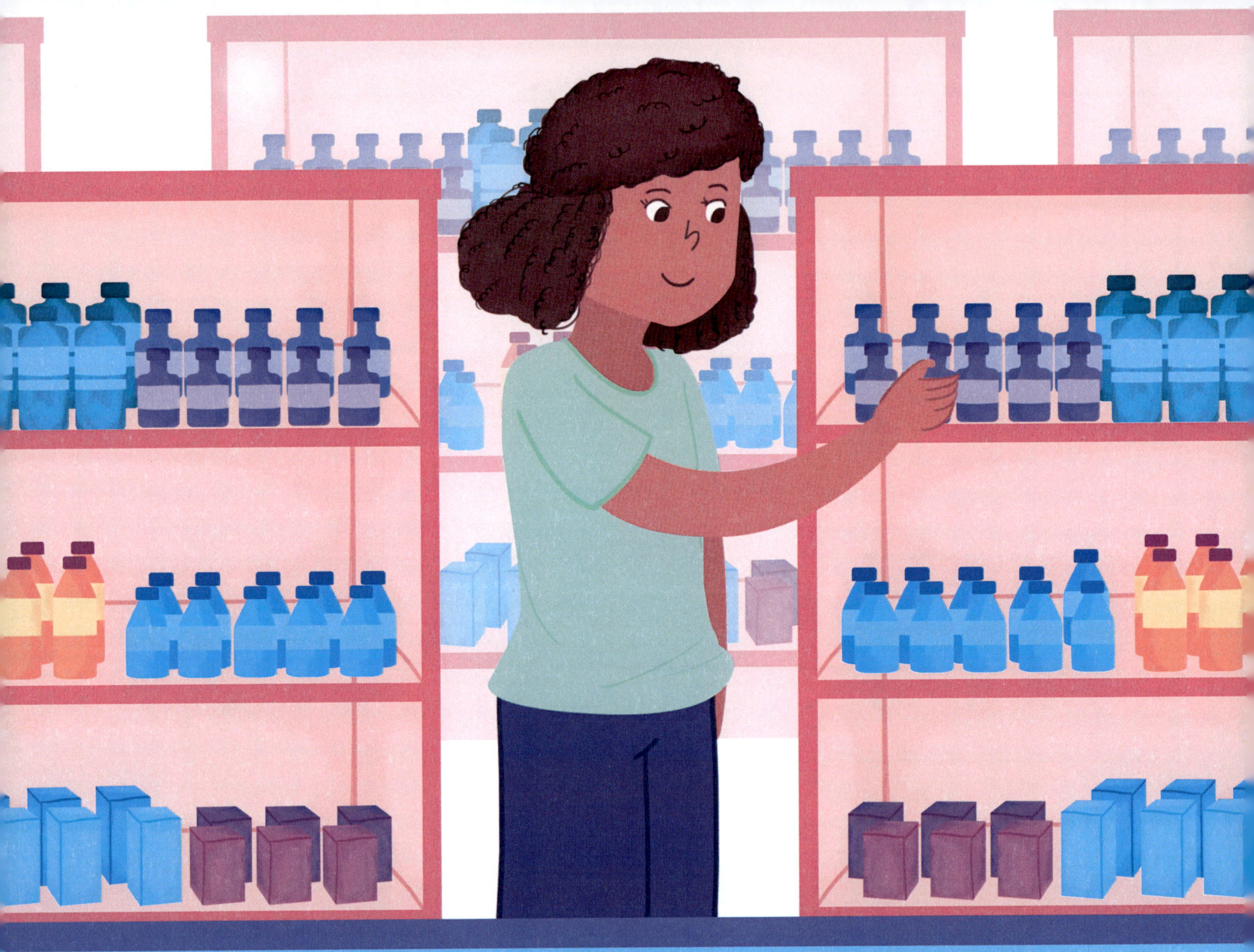

Ibuprofen and acetaminophen are sold **over-the-counter**, which means you don't need a doctor's prescription to buy them.

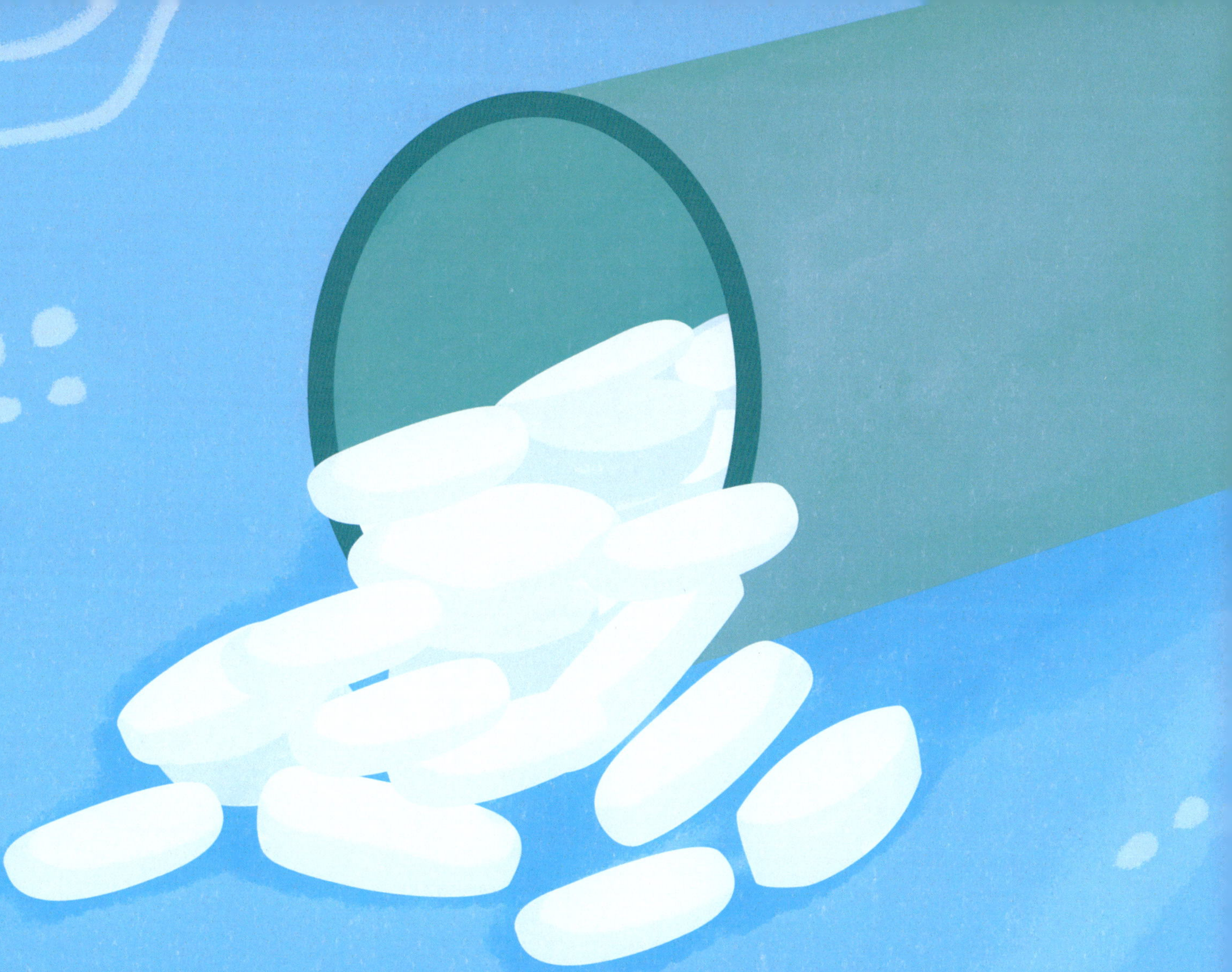

If you are in a lot of pain after surgery, anesthesiologists can prescribe a stronger class of pain medications called **opioids.**

Signs of Opioid Overdose

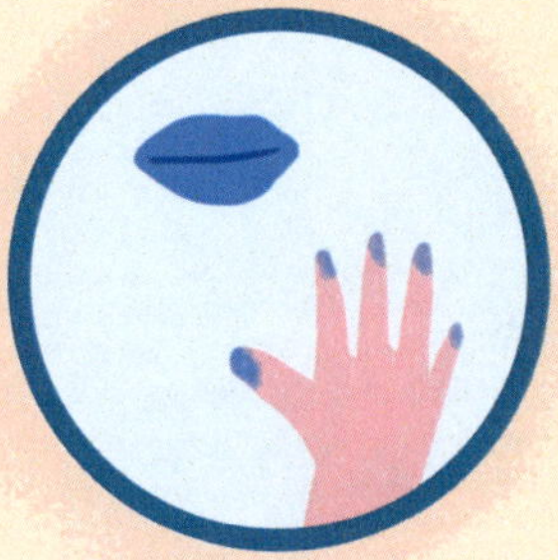

Blue lips
or nails

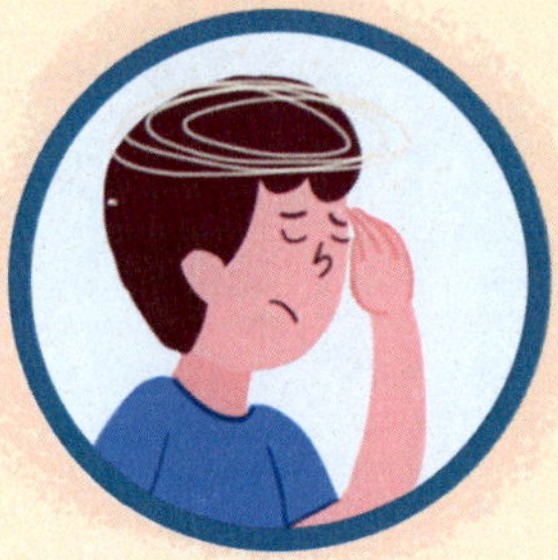

Dizziness and
confusion

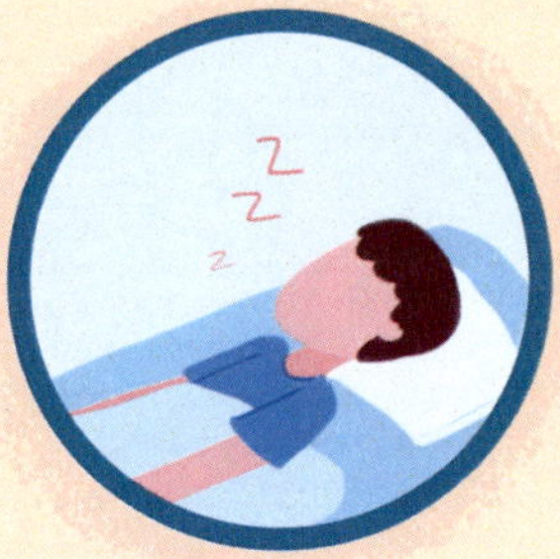

Can't be
woken up

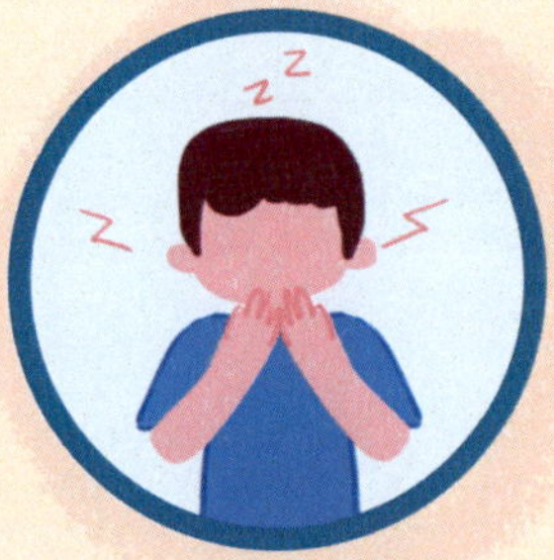

Choking, gurgling
or snoring sounds

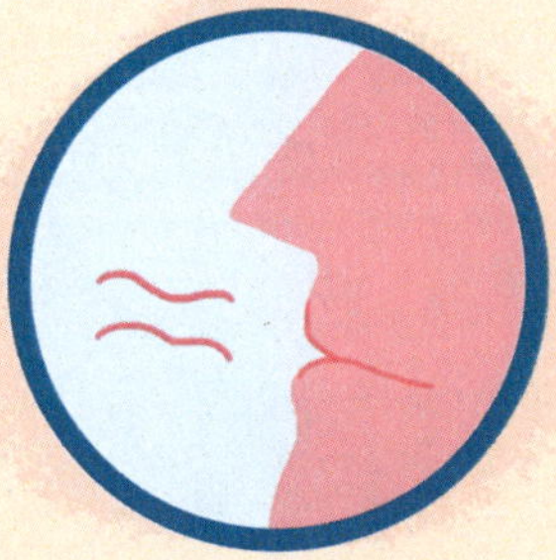

Slow, weak or
no breathing

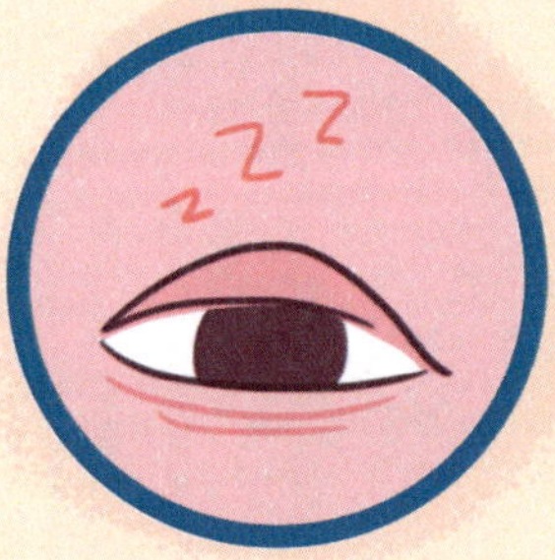

Drowsiness

Opioids are generally safe when used for a short time as prescribed by a doctor, but taking too much can be very dangerous.

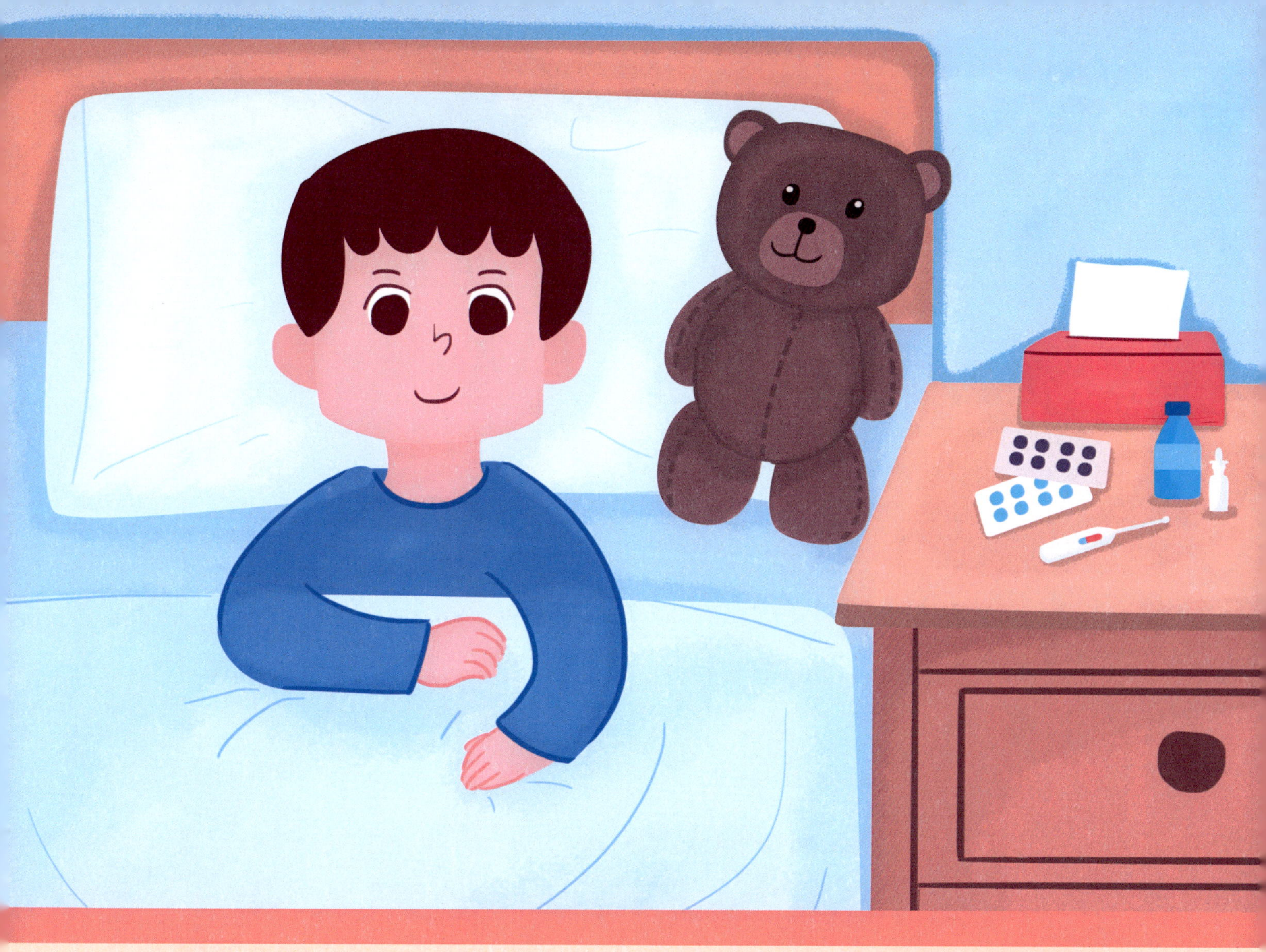

A few days after surgery, you will probably start to feel better. Remember to take it easy! Your body needs time to rest.

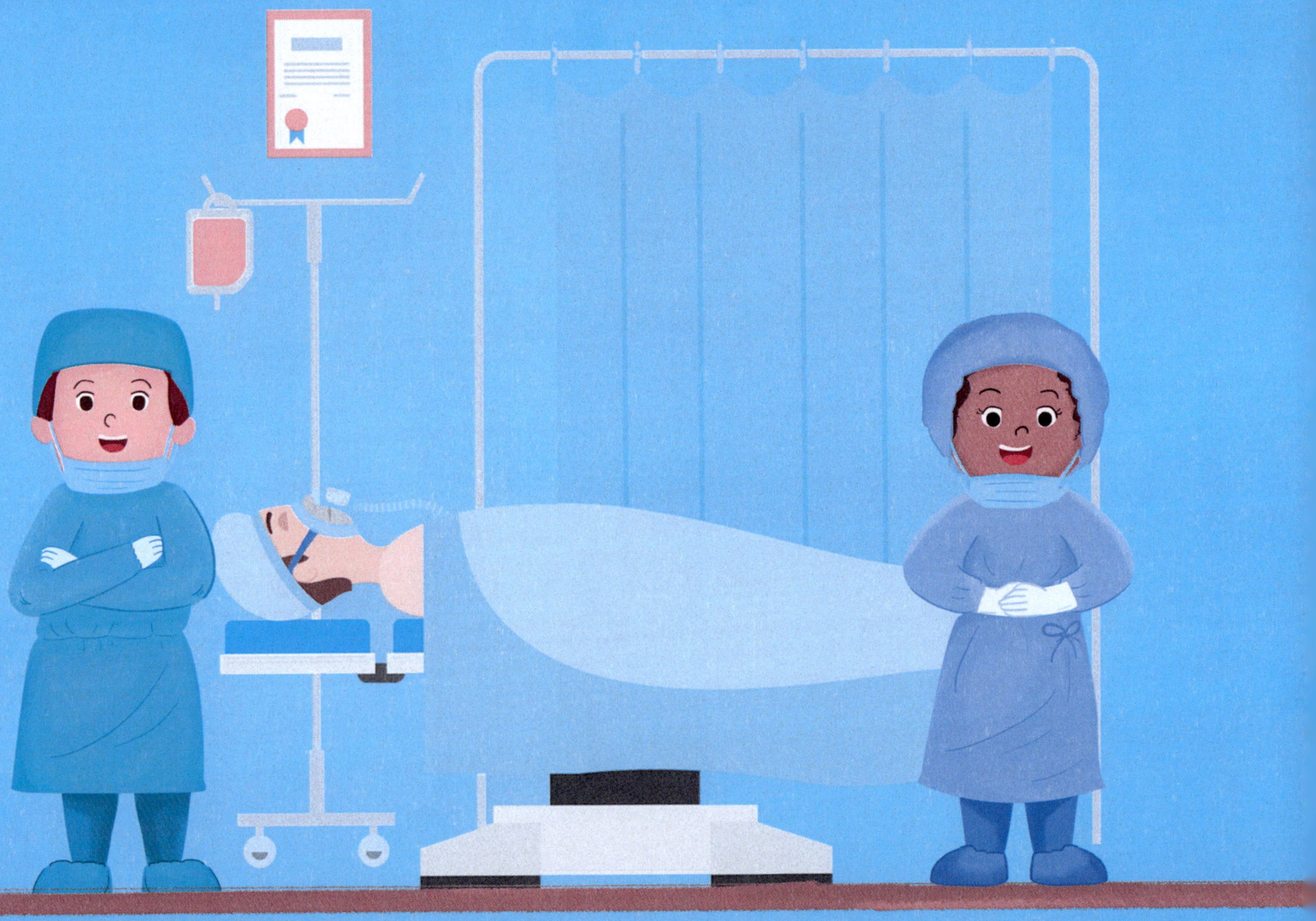

YOU'RE A FUTURE ANESTHESIOLOGIST!

Glossary

Acetaminophen (uh-see-tuh-MI-nuh-fn): non-opioid analgesic and antipyretic medication used to treat pain and fever

Anesthesia (a-nuhs-THEE-zhuh): type of medication that blocks pain signals from getting to the brain

Anxiolytic (ang-zee-ow-LI-tuhk): type of medication used to relieve anxiety

General anesthesia: type of anesthesia that makes someone "asleep"

Ibuprofen (ai-byoo-PROW-fn): type of non-steroidal anti-inflammatory drug (NSAID) used to treat pain, fever, and inflammation

Intubation (in-too-BEY-shun): process by which an anesthesiologist inserts a tube in your throat to help you breathe during surgery

Local anesthesia: type of anesthesia that numbs a small part of the body; can be given as an injection, spray, or ointment

Mechanical ventilation: process by which a machine, called a ventilator, helps bring air in and out of a patient's lungs

Opioids (OW-pee-oydz): class of strong pain medications that require a doctor's prescription; taking too much opioids can be very dangerous

Pain: sensation that you may feel when a part of your body is hurting

Post-anesthesia care unit: location that you are taken to after surgery

Regional anesthesia: type of anesthesia that numbs an entire region of the body; often given as an injection near a cluster of nerves in the spine

Vital signs: clinical measurements that indicate the health of essential body functions (e.g. temperature, heart rate, breathing rate, blood pressure)

Let's review what you learned!

1. What is pain? When does it occur, and what is its function?
2. What type of medication blocks pain signals from getting to the brain?
3. What are the three main types of anesthesia?
4. If you will be getting general anesthesia before a surgery, are you allowed to eat or drink before your surgery? Why or why not?
5. What two types of doctors will you usually see before your surgery?
6. What type of medication might your anesthesiologist give you before your surgery to help you stay calm?
7. What type of people might you meet in the operating room? What will they be wearing and why?
8. What is the process by which an anesthesiologist inserts a tube in your throat to help you breathe during surgery called?
9. What is this breathing tube connected to? What is the process by which this machine helps you bring air in and out of your lungs called?
10. What are some examples of your vital signs?
11. What location do you go to after your surgery?
12. What are two examples of pain medications commonly used after surgery?
13. What is a stronger type of pain medications that requires a prescription?

Medical School FOR KIDS™

Your Answers

1. ______________________________
2. ______________________________
3. ______________________________
4. ______________________________
5. ______________________________
6. ______________________________
7. ______________________________
8. ______________________________
9. ______________________________
10. ______________________________
11. ______________________________
12. ______________________________
13. ______________________________

Answer Key

1. Sensation that we may feel when a part of our body is hurting; can occur when we are sick; functions to tell our body that something may be wrong
2. Anesthesia
3. Local, regional, and general anesthesia
4. No, because having food or water in our stomach can make it dangerous to get anesthesia
5. Anesthesiologist and surgeon
6. Anxiolytic
7. Nurses, doctors, and technicians; wearing caps, masks, and gowns to prevent them from spreading germs to you during surgery
8. Intubation
9. Breathing machine (ventilator); mechanical ventilation
10. Temperature, heart rate, breathing rate, and blood pressure
11. Post-anesthesia care unit (PACU)
12. Ibuprofen and acetaminophen
13. Opioids

Medical School FOR KIDS™

About the Authors

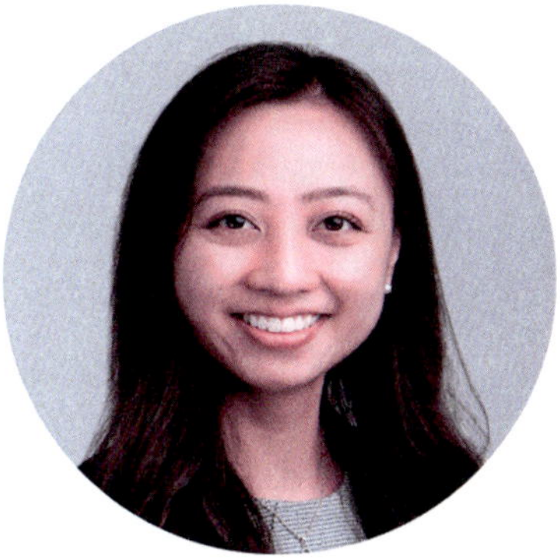

Betty Nguyen

Betty Nguyen was born in California but spent much of her childhood in Georgia, where she grew up on a chicken farm. She received a bachelor's degree in Biology from UCLA, where she received a full-ride Gates Millennium Scholarship through the Bill & Melinda Gates Foundation. Betty also received a full-tuition scholarship to attend medical school at the University of California, Riverside. Outside of work, Betty is a certified yoga instructor and licensed scuba diver. She also enjoys journalistic writing, cycling, and walking her two dogs in her free time.

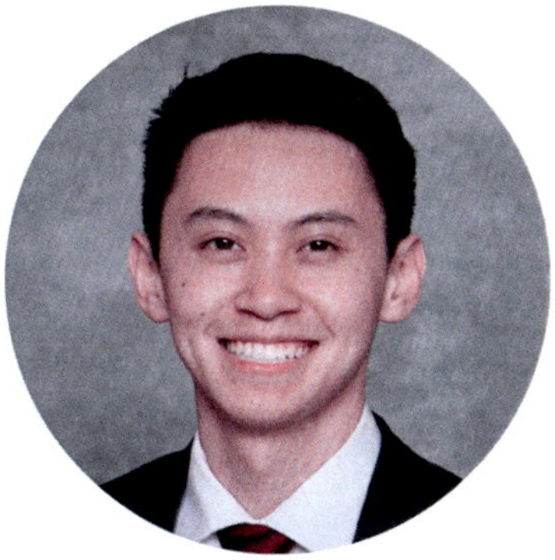

Brandon Pham

Brandon Pham was born and raised in California. He received a bachelor's degree in Microbiology, Immunology, and Molecular Genetics from UCLA, where he was a national Goldwater Scholar. He graduated from Stanford Medical School and is currently completing his residency in ophthalmology at the Bascom Palmer Eye Institute in Miami, Florida. Brandon spent many years teaching for several national test-preparation companies and is passionate about medical education for students of all ages. In his free time, Brandon enjoys traveling, playing tennis, and distance running.

Check out the rest of the books in our series!

Website: mdforkids.org

Instagram: @md.for.kids

Medical School FOR KIDS™

Made in United States
Orlando, FL
04 November 2026

90208507R00024